The Whole Health Manual

A nutrition consultant shows how the body works, what
nutrients it needs ⬛⬛⬛⬛⬛⬛⬛⬛⬛⬛⬛⬛⬛⬛⬛⬛ ⬛day's
unavoidable hazards, ⬛⬛⬛⬛⬛⬛⬛⬛⬛⬛⬛⬛⬛⬛⬛ f health
way bey⬛⬛⬛

THE
WHOLE HEALTH
MANUAL

The comprehensive guide to nutrition and better health

by

Patrick Holford

Illustrated by Christopher Quayle

Thorsons
An Imprint of HarperCollinsPublishers

Thorsons
An Imprint of Grafton Books
A Division of HarperCollins*Publishers*
77-85 Fulham Palace Road,
Hammersmith, London W6 8JB

Published by Thorsons 1981

5   7   9   11   13   15   14   12   10   8   6   4

British Library Cataloguing in Publication Data

Holford, Patrick
The whole health manual. — 3rd ed.
1. Man. Health. Effects of. On diet
I. Title
613.2

ISBN 0-7225-1682-7

Printed in Great Britain by
William Collins Sons & Co. Ltd. Glasgow

Dedication

This book is dedicated to you –
the promoter of your own health.

CONTENTS

FOREWORD

Having spent many years in hospital practice followed by eight years in the pharmaceutical industry I enthusiastically prescribed all the latest medicines. The more drugs I prescribed, the more patients I saw and the more patients I saw, the more drugs I prescribed. I paid little attention to nutrition until I attended a meeting of the McCarrison Society. I then began to look much more closely into the field of nutrition, and by advising patients accordingly, the morbidity in my practice began to fall very significantly. I made further progress when I accompanied the advice with a persuasion to stop smoking.

This new and expanded manual gives guidance in the field of nutrition with information on vitamins and their requirements, together with those of mineral supplements.

I am pleased to see so much new material on the prevention of cardiovascular disease, which I am sure is due in no small measure to faulty nutrition, pollution, smoking and lack of exercise. The expanded section on minerals parallels their importance in maintaining correct body chemistry and function.

I thoroughly recommend *The Whole Health Manual* to all those who wish to maintain positive health.

DR HUGH J. E. COX
T.D., M.B., M.R.C.G.P., D.R.C.O.G., D.C.H.

INTRODUCTION

Throughout history there have been periods when our understanding of health care has made quantum jumps. So often there is one man and one theory, which after initial resistance changes the entire course of medicine.

One such man was Louis Pasteur, a French chemist. He discovered that airborne micro-organisms could cause fermentation and disease. In 1880 he started vaccinating people with micro-organisms relating to particular diseases and found that immunity to that disease resulted. It was then we began pasteurizing our milk, sterilizing our environment and refining our foods.

I believe we are again witnessing the birth of a new age in medicine. No longer does the passive notion of viruses and germs acting upon us sound so plausible. In the same century the father of homoeopathy, Hahnemann demonstrated this in front of a team of eminent physicians. He swallowed enough diptheria virus to kill the entire population of London and did not die! Likewise recent work on vitamin C and vitamin A illustrates that we are not passive organisms in the control of bugs and germs, but that we can achieve total resistance if our health is good. We only attract infection if we are already out of balance, and that infection may have a cleansing effect on us, like a cold which promotes the release of toxic material through the mucus. In other words, *we*, not the germs and viruses, are responsible for our health and lack of it.

Pasteur's works emerged in a time when epidemics were common and as a result of his brilliant work many thousands of people's lives were saved. Yet, in the western world we are no longer threatened by typhoid and cholera. Our primary concerns are the degenerative diseases like cancer, heart disease, rheumatism and arthritis. And we are right to be concerned. After all, 98 per cent of British people will have some form of arthritis before they reach 70, every fifth person who falls sick is taken ill with cancer, and two thirds of men over 45 will die of circulatory disease. In short, only 28 people out of 100, between age 21 and 64, do not have an illness, despite the many thousand million pounds we are spending on health care!

The alarming increase in degenerative diseases has accompanied a drastic change in our lifestyle. The food we eat has changed, the lives we lead are different and probably faster, the air we breathe is polluted. Over 2000 new foods have been introduced in the last hundred years. How do you know what effect they have on us?

Yet there is a danger of making these things the 'germs' of today, the baddies that govern our life, and once more we will end up not responsible for our health. It is the intention of this book to help you to understand your body, how it works, what nutrients it needs, and how it can combat some of today's unavoidable hazards, and most of all to offer you a level of health way beyond normal expectations.

Most medical care has become impersonal, and often concerned solely with treating the symptoms. A holistic approach to health is aimed primarily at understanding the individual as well as finding the cause for any imbalances. It considers all illness to be a necessary part of getting healthier in mind, body and spirit; that colds, fevers, and stomach upsets are the body's way of eliminating toxic material and harmful bacteria; that degenerative diseases such as arteriosclerosis and some forms of cancer only occur when we are abusing our bodies nutritionally or not resolving our mental and emotional problems. The process of getting healthy therefore becomes the process of understanding our body's limits and understanding ourselves.

You are unique

The first and foremost principle of holistic healing is that you are unique. You and I do not have the same face, the same personality, the same ability to produce enzymes, nor the same nutritional needs. We are born different and our life experiences have shaped us differently. For this reason there cannot be one diet, one recommended level of vitamins, protein, and minerals for all people. Our needs are as different as our noses!

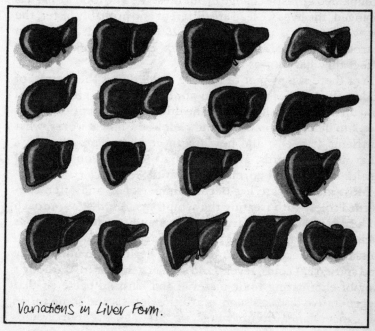

Variations in Liver Form.

Figure 1

Yet common belief contradicts this fact. We are led to believe that all our organs are in the same place, are the same size, produce the same enzymes and need the same nutrients. This simply isn't so.

For instance, livers vary in size as much as 400 per cent. The positioning of the liver is entirely different for each of us. In 4 per cent of the population it all lies behind the ribs on the right side. In 10 per cent of the population it is nearly all below the level of the front ribs (see Figure 2). Individual variations are not just anatomical. We also have unique abilities to make enzymes, which are the chemicals used in digestion. Here again, some of us can produce four times as many enzymes as others. This will have a considerable effect on our ability to use

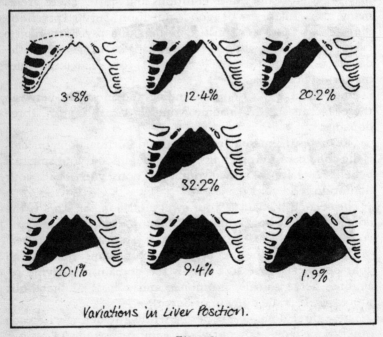

Variations in Liver Position.

Figure 2

the nutrients in the food we eat. Not surprisingly, variations in individual needs for vitamins and minerals are frequently two fold, and often more.

Most of these individual variations concern the variability in efficiency of various physiological systems. In other words some of us will have difficulty digesting fats, while others will have difficulty digesting certain types of protein. However, we still have the same organs (even though the size varies) and the same physiological processes (even though our efficiency varies), and we obey the same nutritional laws.

Nutrition in perspective

The second principle of holistic medicine concerns the interplay between body, mind, emotions and spirit. There are as many case histories of good nutrition curing psychotic illnesses, as there are spiritual healers and psychotherapists curing physical conditions like arthritis or cancer. And the debate which ensues usually tries to prove that mind rules matter or vice versa.

One useful way of understanding the interplay between these factors is to imagine yourself consisting of three domains.

The first is the mental, emotional and spiritual domain. This is the domain of your feelings, your thoughts and your spiritual beliefs. Here are contained your aspirations, your ideals, your limitations and your fears.

The second domain is your structural domain. This is the domain of your bones, muscles, organs – your anatomy and your substance. This is the domain of posture and exercise.

The third area is the chemical domain. It is concerned with all your chemical processes. This is the domain of enzyme reactions, nerve signals, hormones and a host of metabolic processes. It is the domain of nutrition.

These three domains are permanently interacting with each other. If we feel happy our posture improves and so does our

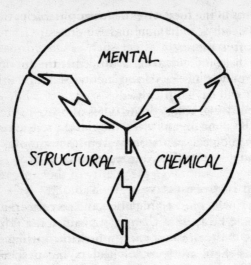

Figure 3

ability to use nutrients. On the other hand if we lack vitamin C
we feel depressed and our posture goes to pieces.

Nutrition and the mind

It is not possible to completely separate mental processes from
nutrition, because every thought or feeling is a physiological
event. When we are afraid our bodies react by producing the
hormone adrenalin. When we are happy a different chemical
change takes place. Likewise other nutrients affect our mental
and emotional state.

For instance B vitamins, which are needed to maintain a
healthy nervous system and hormone balance have been shown
to prevent types of mental illness. In the 1930s it was discovered that pellagra, a disease which causes dementia,
accounted for many of the patients in mental hospitals in the
southern states of America. It was miraculously cured by giving
niacin, vitamin B_3. Drs Osmond and Hoffer have since reported

equally astounding recoveries of schizophrenic patients taking B vitamins and vitamin C in massive doses.

If these nutrients can affect such severe forms of mental imbalance it is not surprising to find that the food we eat will help determine our moods and mental stability.

Nutrition, posture and exercise

The role of exercise, especially in relation to the condition of the respiratory and circulatory systems is now well known, and serves as an illustration of the importance of exercise for good health. Exercise improves the quality of the muscles, it stimulates digestive processes, strengthens blood vessels, heart and lungs, improving blood circulation and oxygen transfer to the cells. Also, even a slight change in posture can improve lung capacity, circulation, and energy flow through the body. In short, posture and exercise help the oxygen in the air and the nutrients in our food to nourish our bodies, as well as loosen up our joints and muscles.

A holistic approach to health must therefore bear in mind the importance of posture and exercise, as well as the effects of mental and emotional stability when balancing nutrition. Only by doing this are you able to reach the highest levels of health in the shortest amount of time.

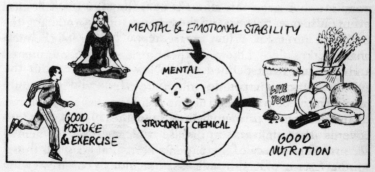

Figure 4

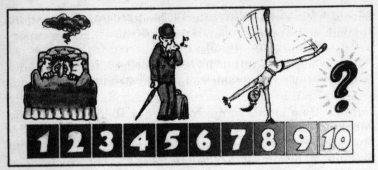

Figure 5

Perfect health is beyond your expectations

The third principle of holistic medicine is that perfect health is a direction and not a goal. Most people have defined health as a lack of illness. The goal of medicine therefore stops once no sign of illness remains. This establishes a norm which we call health. The norm currently includes three colds a year, life expectancy of 70, signs of arthritis after 50 and a Systolic blood pressure of 100 plus your age. Even when research shows us that three colds a year and a life expectancy of 70 is a gross underestimation of our potential, most people remain unconcerned because they believe it is normal. The same is true with pulse rates. A pulse rate of 72 is considered normal, yet my wife's pulse rate, my own and those of my friends who have had good nutrition for a few years are all below 62. Who is normal?

Health has been defined by the law of averages, but the average person simply doesn't exist. If he did he would certainly not be healthy.

Health can be defined not as a definite goal, but as a direction towards increasing sense of well-being, energy, vitality and clarity. Imagine a scale from 1 to 10. Define 1 as seriously ill and 5 as our 'norm' of health such as three colds a year. What state of health do you imagine is a 6, 7, 8, 9 or 10? Our ability to reach these high levels of health is naturally hindered by poor nutrition. But perhaps our greatest limitations are those limiting expectations we impose on ourselves.

How would it be with you if you did not age like those around you? Living in a society which expects to die at 70 is a powerful belief which is hard not to accept. Yet as soon as we mentally limit our time in this world we limit our ability to do all the things we want to do. There are perfectly happy and healthy 110 year olds. How many 60 year olds would be content retiring from life if they knew they had another 50 years to go?

1

UNDERSTANDING YOUR BODY

Nutrition can be defined as the process of receiving food which sustains life. So there are two factors involved. There is the food and the process which makes use of the food. Both are dependent on each other and mankind is dependent on both.

The early days of nutrition were mostly concerned with the substance of food and its various components. As food is the passive component which is acted upon by us, the theories generated by the study of foods tended to be passive themselves. They generated diets recommended for all, high protein diets, high fat diets, high carbohydrate diets. They also resulted in recommended amounts of protein, vitamins and minerals, fads on this mineral, then that vitamin. The motto was 'you are what you eat' and unfortunately not all felt better on the new and varied regimes.

Nutrition is an active, dynamic process. It is not static. We are permanently involved in cycles of digestion, absorption and regeneration. No one stage in the cycles can be isolated because each depends on the previous stage. Your ability to use the foods in today's lunch depends upon the absorption of the nutrients in yesterday's dinner. Bearing this in mind, it is not surprising to find that we have unique abilities to make use of different foods. For example, 60 per cent of the world's adult population, particularly black people, cannot digest milk because they cannot break down milk sugar, but their lives are

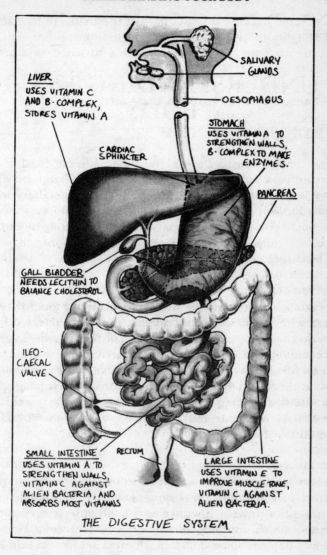

Figure 6

not affected because it is not part of their culture to drink it past babyhood. Also the increasing attention paid to allergies indicates that we should eat according to what we are able to digest.

This section is about your body processes: how it turns food into energy, building material and waste.

THE DIGESTIVE SYSTEM

In the simplest terms we are long tubes. We put food in one end, and pass waste out the other end! What happens in between is a little more complicated. The purpose of digestion is to break down foods into simple units that can pass through our 'inside skin' to nourish our bodies. This is done by various chemicals called enzymes which initiate reactions, changing the food into simpler form.

The mouth

This process starts in the mouth. As we chew our foods they are mixed with saliva, water and ptyalin, which are released from our salivary glands under our tongue. The first enzyme to get to work is ptyalin which breaks down the starch food in grain, into simpler forms of sugar. The salivary juices also make it easier to swallow the food, which is then passed into the oesophagus and moved with a rippling action, known as peristalsis, towards the stomach. As the circular muscle at the top of the stomach relaxes, food enters the stomach.

The stomach

As soon as we place a type of food in our mouth the stomach starts to produce the right enzymes needed to break it down. If the food is a protein it will release hydrochloric acid and an enzyme, which combine to form the first protein digesting enzyme, pepsin. Since the stomach must act like an acid bath its walls are thick and lined with protective mucus secreted by the stomach cells. However, if our diets are continually too acid, or if we don't get enough vitamin A, the wall can break down and ulcers appear.

An excess of acid in the stomach can cause symptoms of heartburn and indigestion, and the usual recommendation is antacids to neutralize the acidity. But, too little acidity will also bring on indigestion because the food is literally in-digested. With the right acid/alkaline balance in the diet, and sufficient vitamins and minerals to help make the enzymes, antacids are not necessary. Since most antacids contain harmful aluminium salts they are best avoided.

Unlike protein, carbohydrates such as potatoes, cannot be digested in such an acid environment. Therefore the stomach doesn't release hydrochloric acid when carbohydrates are eaten. For this reason, some people experience indigestion when eating a concentrated starch and protein. One way round this is to 'stack' your foods and eat the protein first and then the carbohydrate, so that the hydrochloric acid, which is more concentrated in the bottom of the stomach, can work on the protein, leaving the carbohydrate to begin to be digested in the more alkaline part of the stomach. Although food is churned around the stomach, stacking helps the mass of carbohydrate to remain sufficiently alkaline for the ptyalin to act. Some experiments suggest that our stomachs set up a complicated schedule of gastric secretion when presented with foods requiring different enzymes. For instance, when grains are ingested very little acid is released in the first few hours to allow the starch to be completely digested, then acid is released to speed up protein digestion.

The length of time food stays in the stomach depends upon the food. Digestion of fruits and vegetables is completed in under two hours; while starches, proteins, and fats take much longer. A fatty meat may take five hours before it leaves the stomach. The popularity of high fat foods may be a reflection of their long stay in the stomach, creating a well fed sensation.

The partially digested food is then passed from the stomach into the duodenum where the pancreas and gall-bladder secrete their digestive juices for the next stage of the process.

The pancreas

The digestive juices from the stomach are acidic. They trigger the pancreas to release alkaline salts, because the next stage of digestion has to happen in an alkaline medium.

Apart from alkaline salts, the pancreas also produces enzymes to digest fats, proteins and carbohydrates. Unlike the stomach, nothing passes through the pancreas. It merely secretes juices into the duodenum. The 'proteolytic' (protein digesting) enzymes take over where the stomach left off, breaking protein into simpler units, while another enzyme takes over the digestion of starches, breaking it down into maltose, which is a complex sugar. Another enzyme converts the maltose to glucose, and the process is complete, as glucose is the simplest form of sugar and can then be absorbed. In this way starches, which are complex sugars, like bread, are broken down, absorbed, and later used to give us energy. The pancreas is a unique organ because it is not only an organ involved with digestion, but it also acts as a gland, producing hormones which regulate glucose levels.

The gall bladder

The gall bladder stores bile, a substance produced by the liver cells, containing lecithin (pronounced *less-ee-thin*), cholesterol and inorganic salts. When bile is released into the digestive tract this again makes the environment more alkaline. The lecithin in the bile is an emulsifier. Like washing-up liquid, it breaks down fats into smaller units, which can then be acted upon by the pancreatic enzyme lipase. When there is not enough lecithin and too much cholesterol in the bile, gallstones (either cholesterol or calcium deposits) can form. This disrupts fat digestion and can block the bile duct which leads to the duodenum.

The small intestine

Digestion doesn't end as food enters the small intestine. There are still many further enzyme reactions needed before the food is ready to be absorbed. The enzymes released from the pancreas and gall-bladder keep acting, and the small intestine itself produces many more enzymes. Only when carbohydrates become simple sugars, proteins become amino acids, and fats are in small units can absorption take place.

The length of your small intestine is approximately twenty feet, but the surface area is covered with tiny projections called 'villi', and these increase the area available for absorption. If you were to lay out the surface of your small intestine it would be the size of a football pitch! This design ensures maximum contact with nutrients to be absorbed. But, it also means maximum contact with any toxins in the food. The intestinal wall acts as an effective filter, but continued use of irritants like strong spices, drugs and coffee will be harmful. Gluten, a sticky substance found mainly in wheat, and therefore in bread, can

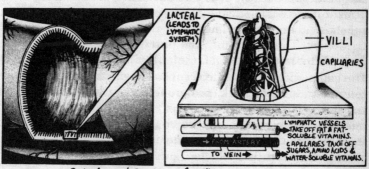

Detail and Section of Villi.

Figure 7

also damage and block up the villi in susceptible people. In cases of bad wheat allergy, the first layer of the villi is literally eaten away. Also, diets consisting of foods that are slow to digest such as meat and fatty foods, can lead to putrefaction and the production of unfavourable bacteria, which disrupt the absorption of nutrients through the intestinal wall.

There is a tendency to think of all bacteria as harmful, but this isn't so. The intestines depend on their 'flora' or garden of beneficial bacteria. Three hundred different strains of bacteria, weighing 3 lb (1½ kg), are present in the large intestine, and a much smaller proportion in the small intestine. These destroy harmful bacteria, neutralizing toxic by-products of digestion, and even manufacture some B vitamins. One way of promoting healthy flora is to eat plenty of yogurt, which contains and promotes the growth of the right bacteria. Yogurt also has the ability to destroy such dangerous organisms as salmonella, typhoid and dysentry. This may be through the effect of lactic acid, in the yogurt, making the environment unfavourable for these virulent microbes. Vitamin C in doses of at least three grams has a similar effect.

The nutrients, now ready for absorption are taken through the outer layer of the villi into the transport systems of the body. Amino acids, sugars, minerals, vitamins, and some fatty substances are taken into the tiny blood vessels called capillaries. These feed into the portal vein which goes to the liver. Other fatty acids and fat soluble vitamins (A, D, E, and K) are taken into the lymphatic vessels which open into the bloodstream in the neck, and are then distributed around the body. The lymphatic vessels form part of a separate transport system to the blood stream, which takes nutrients to the cells. Its main function is to protect against infection, and harmful viruses and bacteria.

Metabolism

Once the nutrients have entered the bloodstream and lymphatic vessels, absorption is complete and metabolism begins. The process of metabolism is the conversion of these nutrients into building materials or energy. Converting nutrients into building material is known as anabolism, and includes the construction of chemicals, hormones, body tissues, enzymes and blood – the stuff we're made of. The conversion of nutrients into energy is called catabolism and takes place by combining oxygen with the breakdown products of glucose and other tissue fuels. The result is energy, carbon dioxide, and water.

The liver

In Chinese medicine the liver is described as the 'minister of planning'. It is concerned with organization and planning for the future.

So it is not surprising to find that its list of functions include the conversion of amino acids from dietary protein, into body protein, the release of glucose to the tissues, the elimination of toxins to the large intestine and kidneys, as well as acting as a short term storage for vitamins, minerals and proteins. So important are its functions that we are born with a liver twice as large in proportion to overall body weight, compared with an average twenty year old. That is why young children look pot bellied – they are carrying around a very large liver.

Protein enters the liver as amino acids. Most of these are reconstructed within the liver to make tissue protein, which is then transported through the blood to be exchanged with old tissue. The remaining amino acids are either stored in the liver or converted into glucose and burned as fuel.

Carbohydrates enter the liver as a simple sugar, such as fructose or glucose. If your diet is balanced most of this is sent out to the body tissues to be used to supply energy. The remainder is stored as glycogen (animal starch) or converted into fat and stored.

Some fats and fat soluble vitamins are supplied direct to the tissues from the small intestine. There the fats are stored, used to make cells, or burnt as fuel. Some are supplied to the liver. These again can be stored as fat or converted into glucose.

People who are deprived of food for a number of days, or athletes who undergo exercise for a long period of time can use up all their stored glucose. They then have to break down fats and protein to produce more glucose. A good example is marathon runners who describe the changeover from carbo-hydrate metabolism to protein metabolism as 'hitting the wall' as it becomes much harder to run, since this is a less efficient way to make energy.

The ileo caecal valve

In the bottom right hand corner of the abdomen, the small intestine feeds what remains of the meal into the large intestine or colon. Between the small and large intestine is a circular muscle, near your appendix, which controls the release of material from one to the other.

This circular muscle is called the ileo caecal valve and although it is a very small part of our anatomy it plays a crucial role. When this valve is functioning correctly it opens up, releasing material into the large intestine, in co-ordination with the stomach releasing material into the small intestine. This action ensures one way traffic, keeping the waste material in the colon. Sometimes the ileo caecal valve stays too open, allowing waste material and bacteria to filter back into the small intestine where they can putrefy and be reabsorbed. This condition is called ileo caecal valve syndrome and is one many of us are likely to encounter. It often originates during a period of stress, which disrupts our proper digestion, putting co-ordination of this valve out of balance. It can be corrected using a massage-like technique called applied kinesiology. Once the valve has been 'closed' using this technique it is wise to follow a diet which excludes all rough foods such as raw fruits and vegetables, whole grains, nuts and seeds. Also avoid coffee, chocolate, spices like chilli, pepper, paprika and alcohol. This diet is not nutritionally balanced and should only be followed for two weeks to allow the valve to recover proper function. You can eat steamed fish, avocados, bananas, cottage cheese, soups, juices, and yogurt.

The large intestine

The main function of the large intestine is to absorb water and salts, to conserve our body fluid, and dry out the faeces. Bacteria also continue digestion and manufacture some B vitamins for reabsorption. When we consider that the colon or large intestine contains 3 lb (1½ kg) and some 300 strains of bacteria we can sense how important their role must be. The right bacteria maintain the right conditions for a healthy intestinal wall, while the wrong bacteria can provide a constant irritation, and produce extremely toxic substances. The wrong bacteria, coupled with a faulty ileo caecal valve, can lead to self toxification.

The average diet, deficient in raw fruits and vegetables as well as whole grains, often leads to sluggish bowels and intermittent constipation. Coupled with a lack of exercise for the stomach muscles, and chronic constipation could be the result. At this stage laxatives are generally prescribed, but although they do relieve the problem, they also deplete the body of important minerals which are usually absorbed in the large intestine. Vitamin C in doses up to 5 grams is the most effective natural laxative, but the only real cure is to eat a diet containing plenty of fibre and vitamin E, and to exercise the stomach muscles. If you can't sit up slowly from a lying position you could benefit from swimming, keep fit exercises, or simply 5 sit-ups each day. But make sure you use your stomach muscles and do not strain your lower back muscles. One way to avoid straining the lower back is to sit up against a wall and lift your legs off the floor.

To maintain a healthy large intestine it is important to eat a diet high in fibre, which includes fruits and vegetables. Watch out for brown bread as a source of fibre as the gluten can prevent proper digestion in some people. Yogurt is also good for promoting healthy bacteria. Here is a chart (opposite) that will help you to know the foods that are high in fibre. Bear in mind that some foods are easier to eat in large quantities than others and are therefore an easier source of fibre. The optimum fibre intake is probably around 30 grams a day.

When using this chart bear in mind that these foods are eaten in different quantities because of the nature of the food, and therefore the percentage of fibre is not the only criterion to select foods by. For instance, 1 lb (½ kg) of bran is much harder to eat than 1 lb of cauliflower.

RESPIRATION AND CIRCULATION

In Eastern philosophy the 'life force' which sustains us is called 'prana'. There are two sources of prana, one is the air we breathe and the other the food we eat.

In nutrition the principle is the same. Without air we cannot live, and the better we breathe and use the nutrients in the air, the better we feel.

Air consists of 21 per cent oxygen, 79 per cent nitrogen and a tiny portion of carbon dioxide. While nitrogen is a basic constituent required to make protein, we cannot use the nitrogen in the air. We can only use nitrogen trapped by plants. We need air primarily because it is the combination of glucose with oxygen, supplied by the blood, which releases energy. If glucose is our 'fuel', oxygen provides the 'fire' needed to burn it.

Respiration
Oxygen is supplied to the lungs through the nasal passages, larynx, trachea and bronchi, which clean, moisten and warm the air, ready for absorption into the bloodstream. As we inhale, air enters the lungs and goes into air sacs. These air sacs

Fibre content in common foods

Food	Percentage of Dietary Fibre
Bran	44
Dried kidney beans	25
Dessicated coconut	23
Dried figs	18
Almonds	14
Dried prunes	13
Lentils uncooked	12
Split peas	12
Stewed apricots	9
Dried dates	9
Brazil nuts	9
Parsley	9
Wholemeal bread	8
Fresh or frozen peas	8
Raspberries and blackberries	7
Muesli	7
Raisins	7
Broccoli tops	4
Mushrooms	2
Cauliflower	2
Avocado	2
Mushrooms	2
Parsnips boiled	2
Celery	2
Lettuce	1

are surrounded by tiny capillaries which take in the fresh oxygen and exchange it for carbon dioxide, a by-product of burning glucose. As we exhale, carbon dioxide leaves the body and the cycle starts again. Oxygenated blood is then taken via

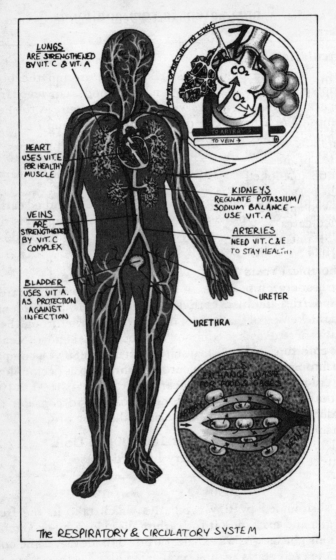

The RESPIRATORY & CIRCULATORY SYSTEM

Figure 8

the capillaries into the pulmonary vein which feeds into the heart.

Circulation

The heart then pumps this fresh blood around the body, supplying the tissues with oxygen. The blood is conveyed from the heart in elastic arteries which change pressure as the heart pumps. The arteries get thinner and thinner until they are miniscule blood vessels called capillaries. At this stage the oxygen and other nutrients in the blood are given up to the body tissues, which in turn give up waste products, carbon dioxide and nutrients.

The blood, having released its oxygen and absorbed carbon dioxide, returns to the heart via the venous system. It is then pumped to the lungs, ready to exchange carbon dioxide for oxygen and begin the cycle again.

Arteriosclerosis

The leading cause of death in the Western world is cardio-vascular disease which includes arteriosclerosis, the hardening and thickening of the walls of the arteries. Death through heart attacks or strokes is so common that society has almost accepted this epidemic as the normal state of affairs. But if you compare the number of deaths from coronary thrombosis (a clot blocking the flow of blood to the heart) over the years 1890 to 1970 in the table below it is no longer possible to consider this epidemic disease as part of the natural ageing process.

Death rates (per 100,000) in USA from coronary heart disease

1890	0*
1950	213
1960	275
1970	340

* (Faulty diagnosis probably contributes to this exceptional figure)

The advances in medicine which have dramatically decreased the number of deaths before the age of twenty, have disguised the fact that once over 50 (the prime time for heart attacks) life expectancy has changed little since 1900! For instance, in 1900 a man aged 65 had a life expectancy of 76.5 years. In 1960 a 65 year old man was expected to live to 77.9. I believe that the disguise of these alarming statistics, have lulled us into a false sense of security about the effects of twentieth century living, eating, food adultery and pollution.

Arteriosclerosis worsens over a number of years and usually follows a sequence. First the inner lining of the artery wall is stripped away, leaving a bare patch. As cells deeper in the wall multiply at these patches, fatty substances, especially cholesterol, eventually accumulate. By this stage the artery is thinner and blood clots (thromboses) can stick to the arterial 'growth', causing a complete blockage.

While we are generally advised to avoid smoking, stress, lack of exercise, and salt, which hardens the arteries, the major cause is said to be high blood cholesterol levels, probably consequent to a diet high in saturated fat mainly from animal food sources. This has been the general view since 1950 but it has not made any appreciable difference to the severity and frequency of this disease.

We now know that arterial deposits are not just the result of too much cholesterol floating around in the blood, and sticking to the walls. The process of forming arterial deposits is complex and probably starts by chemicals called free radicals damaging the artery wall causing the proliferation of cells within the artery, much like the proliferation of cancer cells. The damaged artery wall can't keep cholesterol (and other fats) out so cells become engulfed with fat and form a porridge-like build up that narrows the artery and raises blood pressure. However, artery deposits alone do not cause heart attacks. The other condition needed is, put simply, sticky blood. Thick blood can then form a clot at the point where the artery has become narrow due to arterial deposits, depriving the heart or brain of blood.

Preventing heart disease

Of course, knowing how arterial deposits form in the first place gives us insight into how to read the early warning signals and take effective action. Certainly one thing that has become clear as a result of many millions of pounds spent researching this condition is that there is no one cause, but a multitude of con-tributive factors. For example, smoking alone may not be enough to cause heart disease, but smoking, eating too much sugar and fats, and leading a stressful life may add up to heart disease even though none are done to excess.

Smoking

Smoking is one addiction that has become far more of a problem in this century. As any regular smoker knows, break-ing the nicotine habit is far from easy. Some research suggests that most people (98 per cent) are susceptible to nicotine addiction, and can become hooked after as little as a cigarette a day for fourteen days.

According to one research study by the American Heart Association, smokers increase their risk of heart attack by 70 per cent. A man aged 25 can expect to live 6.5 years longer than a 'packet a day' smoker. The reasons that smoking is so dangerous for the health of the respiration and circulation system are many.

Firstly, cigarettes contain a toxin called benzopyrene which can trigger off the proliferation of cells in the arteries. Secondly, smoking increases your chances of a blood clot since it interferes with the body's ability to dissolve clots. Coupled with the fact that nicotine is a constrictor of blood vessels, a cigarette is enough to tip the balance for someone who already has a degree of arteriosclerosis and clots in the blood.

The smoker is also less likely to survive a heart attack since

The following questionnaire is designed to let you assess how you rate on each of the major risk factors The central diagram represents the diameter of an artery. For each point you score, shade in one of the blocks starting at the outside, to see at a glance your risk of heart disease. The greater the risk the smaller the diameter of the artery, giving less room for the blood to flow and a higher risk of blockages.

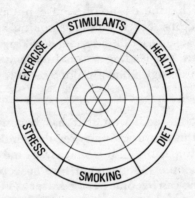

Stimulant Check

Colour in one section in the stimulant sector for every YES answer

a) Do you drink more than four cups of coffee a day?
b) Do you drink more than six cups of tea a day?
c) Do you have more than three alcoholic drinks a day?
d) Do you often eat chocolate more than three times a week?
e) Do you add sugar to food or drink every day?

Health Check

Colour in one section in the health sector for each YES answer

a) Is your pulse over 90 beats per minute?
b) Have you ever had high blood pressure?
c) Have either of your parents had high blood pressure or diabetes?
d) Is there a broader family history of heart disease or diabetes?

Diet Check
Colour in one section in the diet sector for every YES answer

a) Do you use salt when cooking and add it to your food?
b) Do you eat fried food more than twice a week?
c) Do you eat white bread or rice and processed foods more than whole grains, lentils or beans?
d) Do you eat red meat. more than twice a week?
e) Does less than a third of your diet consist of raw fruit and vegetables?

Stress Check
Colour in one section in the stress sector for each YES answer

a) Do you feel guilty when relaxing?
b) Do you have a persistent need for recognition or achievement or are you especially competitive?
c) Do you work harder than most or do you often do two or three tasks at a time?
d) Do you easily become angry or impatient if things hold you up?
e) Do you find it difficult to openly admit defeat?

Smoking Check
Colour in one section in the smoking section for each YES answer

a) Do you smoke 1–10 cigarettes a day?
b) Do you smoke more than 10 cigarettes a day?
c) More than 15?
d) More than 20?
e) Do you smoke a pipe or cigars?

Exercise Check
Colour in one section in the exercise sector for each NO answer

a) Do you take exercise that noticeably raises your heartbeat for more than 20 minutes, three or more times a week?
b) Does your job involve lots of walking, lifting or vigorous activity?
c) Do you regularly play an active sport?
d) Do you have any physically tiring hobbies?
e) Do you consider yourself to be fit?

smoking destroys the tiny air sacs in the lungs, starving the body of oxygen. The ability to get oxygen through to the heart both during and after a heart attack helps to speed up the healing process.

How to stop smoking

Every smoker gets bored of hearing how terrible the habit is and has first hand experience of its damaging effects to the health. In fact, a large majority of Britain's 22 million smokers would love to quit but the question is how.

Smokenders, an organization set up in 1969, run a series of eight evening seminars, one a week, to help people kick the habit. They have a genuine 75 per cent success rate for people stopping smoking and still not smoking a year later, and on five-year follow-up studies over 50 per cent don't smoke. People who complete the course simply have no desire to smoke, they don't put on weight or have a tough time giving up – they just give up. Over 250,000 people have completed the courses in America including America's former Secretary of Health.

There are a number of reasons why Smokenders, called Habit Breakers in England, works and one of them is that they identify the habitual triggers which go with smoking. For instance many people smoke after a meal, a cup of coffee, when the phone rings, in a business meeting and so on. Until these smoking habits are broken, the person who attempts to give up is confronted with a multitude of habits, and a multitude of smoking habits which wear down even the strongest resolve. Habit Breakers can be contacted by calling 081-968 6807. Their director, Simon Morgan, has also written an excellent book *How to Stop Smoking* published by Virgin Books (1987).

Sugar

Sugar is another contributive factor to heart disease. Firstly, refined sugar uses up stores of B_6 and chromium which are essential for a healthy heart and arteries. It also makes the blood more 'sticky', acts as an adrenal stimulant and encourages diabetes which is known to lead to heart disease.

The antioxidants – C, E and selenium

One of the factors that can trigger cell proliferation is the presence of 'free radicals' which are dangerous oxides, created as the body uses oxygen. These dangerous by-products are rendered harmless by anti-oxidant enzyme systems and anti-oxidant nutrients. The three most important nutrients are vitamins C, E and selenium.

Vitamin C not only protects against cell proliferation but it is also an effective nutrient for reducing blood clotting. Vitamin E has much the same effect and also has the added bonus of lowering blood pressure.

Areas where the selenium soil level is high have fewer deaths through heart disease, and unfortunately most of Britain has fairly low levels of this mineral. Selenium works with vitamin E and has much the same effect.

Balancing your fats

The current trend of eating masses of polyunsaturated fats and little cholesterol has the potential of doing more damage than good. An excess of total fat has been linked to heart disease, so it is important to be aware of your overall fat intake and the ratio of saturated, animal fats, and polyunsaturates. This is explained in more detail in the section about Fats.

Relaxation and exercise

We are a society geared to work, we are taught how to work and learn few skills to help us relax. Not surprisingly, stresses and unresolved pressures in our lives reflect in our overall health, yet relaxation is as essential to us as sleep. The more you over-work, the more tense you become, the more likely you are to be affected by heart problems. Unfortunately, the trend towards technological advances for manual jobs has also lowered the overall amount of exercise any of us get through work.

Exercise tones the muscles and strengthens the heart. It is important to build up your exercise slowly, so as not to cause strain, however at least an hour of vigorous exercise a week will help to lower your pulse rate and blood pressure. For example, a 30 year old should do exercises which increase their pulse into the range of 140–160 beats per minute. A 65 year old should stay below 130 and above 105 during exercise.

The secret of the Eskimos

Some cultures such as Eskimos, have a diet high in cholesterol and saturated fats but have virtually no heart disease. Dr Hugh Sinclair set out in 1954 to discover why. The answer was EPA, a type of fat that is actually good for the heart.

EPA is a type of essential fatty acid that can be made from vegetable oils but is most abundant in oily fish, the staple diet of the Eskimo. This essential fatty acid does everything to reduce the risk of heart disease. It lowers blood pressure, thins the blood, lowers blood levels of fats, including cholesterol, and stimulates the removal of excess cholesterol from the arteries. This magical fish oil is now being used for the treatment of angina, a condition caused by narrowing of the arteries leading to the heart.

EPA is itself converted in fish from linolenic acid which is found in nuts, seeds, and vegetable oils. The fish get linolenic acid from plankton, and then the large fish eat the small fish, further concentrating EPA and another fat called DHA, which is an important structural component in nerve, and brain cells. We then turn EPA into hormone-like substances called prostaglandins.

Blood pressure

Blood pressure is one of the easiest ways of monitoring the

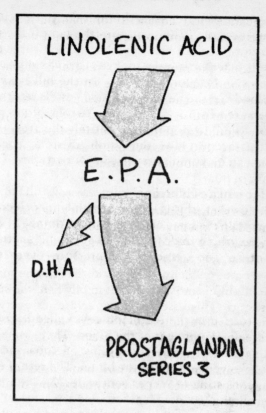

Figure 9

health of your circulation system. It is also easy to do yourself—however, every time you see your doctor you should ask him what your blood pressure is. A 35 year old man with a blood pressure of 120/80 is expected to live 20 years longer than a man with a blood pressure of 150/100. So what do these figures mean, and what should yours be?

The easiest way to visualize what these figures mean is to imagine a hose pipe connected to a water tap: as you turn on the tap, a surge of water goes through the pipe, causing the pressure to increase. When you turn the tap off the pressure returns to zero. As your heart pumps the next surge of blood through your arteries the pressure rises to a maximum, which is called your systolic blood pressure. In the lull between this surge of blood and the next, your blood vessels return to their lowest pressure which is called your diastolic blood pressure. (If the blood were to stop flowing entirely the pressure would be zero.) This is reported as your systolic/diastolic. For example 120/80 means a maximum pressure in your arteries of 120, and a minimum of 80.

The old formula of blood pressure was a systolic of 100 plus your age. However, this is almost certainly incorrect and it is safer to maintain the same blood pressure from age 21 onwards. Generally, anything under 120/80 is good and anything over this is not so good, and blood pressure over 160/95 is serious.

Blood
Oxygen is carried in the red blood cells called haemoglobin, which make up 45 per cent of the blood. There are also white blood cells which act as a defence against bacteria, and platelets which are involved in clotting the blood. The rest of the blood is plasma, consisting of 90 per cent water.

The remaining 10 per cent of blood plasma consists of proteins, as well as vitamins, minerals and waste products such as carbon dioxide and uric acid. Some of the proteins form antibodies which are important for our immunity against viruses. Others form hormones, the chemical messengers in our body.

Vitamins and minerals are taken to the cell sites where they are used or stored, while waste products are expelled through the lungs, skin, in the bile, or the kidneys.

Kidneys
The kidneys are organs of elimination. They filter the blood,

removing most of the toxic by-products left after burning glucose, and a host of other unwanted substances. These are passed out of the body in the urine. The kidneys play an important role in maintaining the right alkaline balance of the blood and body fluids.

The filtration process takes place because the pressure in the arteries within the kidneys is so great as to force fluid through the artery wall. This fluid consists largely of water and also glucose, salt, urea, potassium, phosphates and sulphates. Much of this is later reabsorbed back into the blood.

The kidneys reabsorb a high proportion of glucose and salt, and a low proportion of potassium. With the increasing evidence that the 'average' Western diet contains too much salt and a lack of potassium, it may be surprising to see the kidneys reabsorbing salt.

A brief look at history may reveal the answer. Through the many generations that mankind relied more heavily on fruits and vegetables for sustenance, potassium was readily available and salt was not.

For this reason we may have adapted to retain salt, and release potassium as it was readily available. However, in the last 100 years the situation has reversed. Our intake of salt has increased tremendously and potassium levels in the soil are low. Our bodies have not changed as fast as our diets and the excess use of salt is increasing the incidence of hypertension, arteriosclerosis and kidney disease.

Apart from decreasing salt intake and drinking plenty of water, getting an adequate intake of vitamin A helps to strengthen the kidneys.

THE CONTROL SYSTEMS

All the different processes and stages of digestion, absorption, metabolism, and elimination are carefully co-ordinated events. So is the cycle of respiration, and the functions of the circulation system involving the heart, lungs, and kidneys. All these events are scheduled and controlled by the brain, nervous system and endocrine glands.

The nervous system and endocrine glands are also intimately involved with our moods. As our mood changes, or if we are under stress, change takes place throughout our nerves and glands. They are the meeting point between mind and body.

The central nervous system

The nervous system is a vast electrical network. It can be divided into two parts: the central nervous system and the autonomic nervous system. The central nervous system includes the brain and spinal cord, and it is here that our mental processes, creative thoughts, imagination and judgement take place. It is through this system that we interpret the information from our senses. We can then send messages down the spinal cord which activate movements. The incredible ease with which we can perform such complex functions is something we all take for granted.

The autonomic nervous system

The autonomic nervous system is so named because generally speaking it controls functions that are not normally under conscious control. However, certain functions like blood pressure and heart rate can be easily altered through biofeedback techniques. Biofeedback, as the name implies, involves giving feedback regarding some life (bio) process. For example, by monitoring his nervous activity a person can consciously quieten it by inducing relaxation. In this way an autonomic function becomes consciously altered. Perhaps all that is needed to consciously alter any autonomic function is awareness, which can come through feedback of that function. If this is so, it suggests that the conscious direction of thought towards healing any illness in the body can have a positive effect.

The autonomic nervous system is divided into the parasympathetic and sympathetic nervous system. Both these systems have their highest centres in the brain and co-ordinate the functioning of the organs, working in opposition. Stimulation of the parasympathetic nerves encourages vegetative functions in the body, such as the peristaltic motion of the intestines, and the slowing of the heart rate. On the other hand, stimulating the sympathetic nerves appears to get the body ready for emergencies. The heartbeat goes up, digestion stops and hormones involved with increasing availability of glucose, thus energy, are released. The maintenance of stable body processes is helped by the opposing actions of these two parts of the autonomic nervous system.

Endocrine glands

Higher brain centres, most notably the hypothalamus, influence the endocrine glands, which also regulate body processes.

Pituitary

The pituitary gland, situated in the centre of the head at eye level, is called the 'master gland' because it controls all other glands and forms the link between the nervous system and the glands, via the hypothalamus. In addition any imbalance with the adrenal glands, thyroid and parathyroid glands or sex glands will affect and be affected by the pituitary. Because of its central role it is important to maintain the fine balance of the hormones it produces. These hormones are chemical messengers which stimulate the other glands. So, while the nervous system sends electrical messages, the endocrine gland system communicates through chemical messages.

One part of the pituitary gland stimulates the thyroid, adrenal and sex glands, and the hormone which encourages growth of body tissues. The posterior part stimulates the kidneys and tissues to retain water (this happens when there is a lack of dietary water, or a loss through excess sweating, or

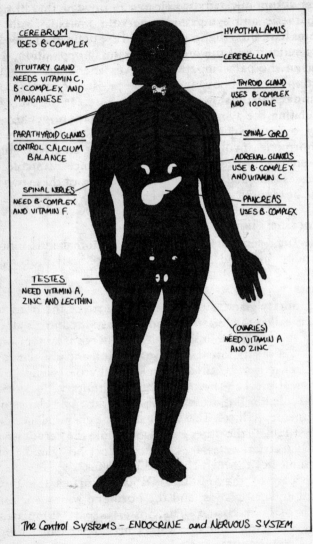

CEREBRUM
USES B·COMPLEX

HYPOTHALAMUS

CEREBELLUM

PITUITARY GLAND
NEEDS VITAMIN C,
B·COMPLEX AND
MANGANESE

THYROID GLAND
USES B·COMPLEX
AND IODINE

PARATHYROID GLANDS
CONTROL CALCIUM
BALANCE

SPINAL CORD

ADRENAL GLANDS
USE B·COMPLEX
AND VITAMIN C

SPINAL NERVES
NEED B·COMPLEX
AND VITAMIN F.

PANCREAS
USES B·COMPLEX

TESTES
NEED VITAMIN A,
ZINC AND LECITHIN

(OVARIES)
NEED VITAMIN A
AND ZINC

The Control Systems – ENDOCRINE and NERVOUS SYSTEM

Figure 10

excess dietary salt). It also releases a hormone that brings on uterine contractions and encourages the release of milk from the breast after birth. To perform all these functions properly the pituitary needs adequate vitamin B complex, C and manganese.

The adrenals

Demanding jobs, near car crashes, sugar, salt, cigarettes,

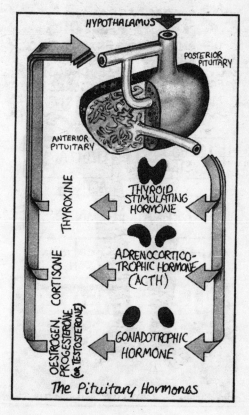

Figure 11

coffee, and alcohol all have one thing in common: they stress our bodies and stimulate the release of adrenal hormones. First an electrical message releases adrenalin, and later a chemical messenger, ACTH, is sent from the pituitary to the adrenals which then release cortisone.

These two adrenal hormones get us ready for action. Blood sugar levels go up, heartbeat goes up and blood pressure increases to get oxygen and sugar to the cells for energy

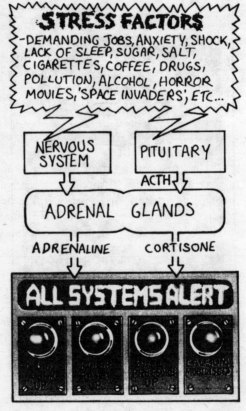

Figure 12

production. We stop digesting and pour all necessary nutrients into the nerves and muscles so we are ready to act fast.

Adrenal exhaustion

Normally the need for this reaction ends and we reverse the process. However, continued stress will rob us of nutrients, slow down digestion, and weaken our resistance to infection. In the long run the situation is even worse. Prolonged adrenal stimulation leads to adrenal exhaustion. As well as the above symptoms one can expect a tendency to put on weight, heightened blood cholesterol levels, slower thought processes and less energy.

The more exhausted our adrenals get the more stimulants are needed to get an energy response. We literally become addicted to the foods which do us most damage.

There is only one way out of this vicious cycle, and that is to reverse the process. All stressors must be avoided and a balanced diet, high in nutrients must be followed. However, these factors alone will not restore energy to the owners of exhausted adrenal glands. They also need vitamin B complex, especially B_5, B_3 and lecithin, and vitamin C. By taking these supplements in effective doses a new balance of energy will appear within a few weeks. For best results take these supplements two times a day for a month at breakfast and lunch. Then decrease to once a day.

Thyroid

Stress also affects the thyroid glands which govern our rate of metabolism. The thyroid is stimulated by the pituitary which releases TSH (thyroid stimulating hormone). When this chemical message is released from the pituitary, the thyroid releases hormones which speed up the energy producing processes in the cells. In this way they work with the adrenals to speed us up.

There is a basic law with all glands which is that continued over-stimulation will eventually lead to underfunctioning. So a continued stimulation of the thyroid glands will lead to increased weight, sluggish digestion and slower thought processes.

Parathyroid

The thyroid gland sits in the neck on the side of our trachea, and the parathyroids, which are much smaller, sit behind the thyroid. These glands control the distribution of calcium in the

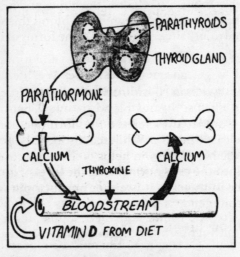

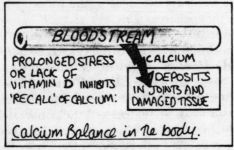

Figure 13

body and therefore play a crucial role in arthritic conditions. Normally, when there is a 'stress' signal from the pituitary the parathyroids release a hormone which stimulates the release of calcium from the bones into the blood. Calcium is needed by the muscles to function properly, so this reaction gets us ready for action. Once the 'stress' signal is over, the thyroid releases a hormone which attracts the calcium back to the bones.

When there is continued stress or a lack of vitamin D which is needed to absorb dietary calcium, the bones and joints become brittle. If there is excess calcium in the blood this will settle in joints and old injury sites resulting in some forms of rheumatism and arthritis.

Pancreas

The pancreas works in co-ordination with the adrenal glands to balance the glucose in our bloodstream. When the adrenal glands are stimulated to release the hormone cortisone, the pancreas releases insulin. While cortisone raises the level of glucose in the blood, insulin helps take the glucose out of the blood and into the cells normalizing the level of glucose in the blood. Once in the cells it is either burnt or put into storage when the emergency is over.

High and low blood sugar

If we continually eat sugar, insulin must be repeatedly released to normalize the level of sugar in the blood. After frequent stimulation the pancreas can get trigger happy and over-produce insulin. The over-compensation results in low blood sugar or hypoglycaemia. It is often caused by adrenal exhaustion. Once our adrenals are getting exhausted we need twice as much sugar to get the same boost of energy. The extra sugar intake can then bring on an overproduction of insulin.

When the adrenals are exhausted the pancreas has to work harder producing insulin. When the pancreas gets worn out and insulin production goes down, blood sugar levels are no longer regulated and high blood sugar, or hyperglycaemia results. Diabetes is a severe form of this. Since the pancreas cannot make its own insulin it becomes necessary to inject it to normalize blood sugar.

Since the adrenals and pancreas are so closely related it is unusual to find stress affecting one and not the other. So most stressed people will have a fluctuating blood sugar level. One day they will be speeding around busily and the next day they'll be exhausted. Other related symptoms are a low resistance to

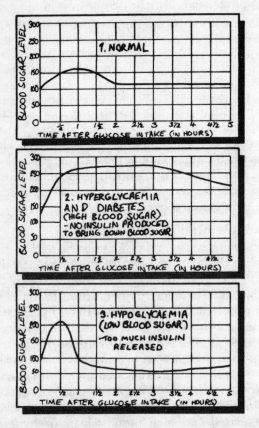

Figure 14

infection, depression, arthritic conditions, and allergies. To restore the pancreas to proper functioning, the adrenals must be supported with B and C vitamins.

The discovery of insulin as an important factor in controlling blood sugar levels happened partly as a result of the discovery that animals without a pancreas become diabetic. However, what has been largely forgotten is that animals without a liver suffer the same fate. While it has been known that there is a substance in the liver which also controls blood sugar levels, it is only recently that this substance was identified as containing the mineral chromium, vitamin B_3 (niacin), and two amino acids. This substance is called Glucose Tolerance Factor, or GTF for short, and helps insulin to be more effective. Every time the blood sugar level goes up GTF is released to help bring it down. However, it seems to have a controlling effect for both hypo and hyperglycaemics. For this reason, supplementation of chromium and B_3 sometimes has astounding results for diabetics and other people who have faulty sugar metabolism.

Since chromium is processed out of refined sugar and grains, a diet high in refined foods leads to chromium deficiency and a lack of GTF. What's more, since GTF is released every time the blood sugar level goes up, and then excreted once it has done its job, the more quick releasing sugars you eat, or the more stressors like coffee, cigarettes, and mental stress that you experience, the more you will use up your GTF reserves. Hair Mineral Analysis reveals the common pattern of low chromium for hypoglycaemics and diabetics. See Nutrition Programmes for Common Diseases, including hypoglycaemia and diabetes.

Histamine – a cause for schizophrenia?

Apart from the many hormones which regulate and balance our glands, there are many other complex substances which are involved in nerve transmission and brain function, which help maintain balanced body chemistry. One of these is histamine, which we usually associate with allergies since most allergic responses are a result of a production of excess histamine.

The discovery that 50 per cent of so called 'schizophrenics' have unusually low levels of histamine, and 20 per cent have unusually high levels of histamine, has led to a breakthrough in the treatment of people suffering with mental disorders such as severe depression, paranoia, hallucinations, obsessions and phobias.

The low histamine type tends to suffer mainly with thought disorders, paranoia, and hallucinations. They usually have high copper, low zinc, and a high pain threshold, as well as lots of dental fillings, and are rarely allergic. The low histamine person responds well to supplementation of vitamin C, B_3, folic acid, B_{12}, zinc and manganese.

The high histamine type tends to be depressed and suicidal, having overriding obsessions and phobias. They usually experience lots of headaches, have a very low pain threshold and produce too much saliva, protecting their teeth against fillings. For these people zinc and manganese are beneficial, but B_{12} and folic acid can worsen symptoms. See the Nutrition Programme for Healthy Minds later in this book.

The immune system

As a result of the AIDS epidemic, more and more is being discovered about the immune system. This is a complex mechanism, consisting of different types of cells that roam our blood and lymphatic system on the look-out for anything that isn't us. This could be a flu virus, a cell that has become cancerous, or even a food particle that has been absorbed in an incompletely digested state. A reaction to a food involving the immune system is called an allergy (more on this later), so cancer, allergies, and frequent infections are all examples of immune diseases. Sometimes the immune system becomes defective in that it starts to destroy its own army of cells. This is what happens in rheumatoid arthritis, known as an auto-immune disease. The immune system needs good nutrition to stay strong. Particularly essential is enough of vitamins A, C, and E, as well as zinc, calcium, magnesium, and selenium.

2

BALANCING YOUR DIET

As the possibility of an oil crisis draws nearer, mankind frantically searches for a form of energy that will meet his needs and not poison his environment. Meanwhile he is unconsciously involved in the biggest energy project and recycling plant that exists. The source of the energy is the sun, and the process of extraction involves the earth, the sea, the sky and all animals, vegetables and minerals.

The conversion of sun energy into energy we can absorb, takes place in the plants. Carbon dioxide in the air and water from the soil and clouds are absorbed by plants. As sunlight strikes the leaves, carbon dioxide and water combine to form carbohydrate, trapping the sun's energy. This process is known as photosynthesis. The only by-product is oxygen, which is given off into the air. Ourselves and animals then eat the carbohydrate and inhale the oxygen. The two combine and the stored energy in carbohydrate is released, in much the same way as the spark releases stored energy in petrol which drives your car. This process is known as catabolism. The only by-products are carbon dioxide and water, which are later re-absorbed by the plant, so completing the energy cycle in nature.

Plants do not consist solely of carbohydrate, they also contain fats and protein. Fats are essentially a different form of carbohydrate, which lends itself more readily to storage in our bodies. When we have no immediate source of carbohydrate to 'burn', we start to break down our fat deposits and burn these instead.

Plants require more than carbon, hydrogen, oxygen, and the sun to make protein. They also need nitrogen and sometimes sulphur or phosphorus. These occur in the soil in the form of nitrates, sulphates, and phosphates. With these ingredients and the light of the sun, the plant can synthesize protein. When we eat plants and sometimes the animals which have eaten plants, we absorb this protein, which is the major constituent of all our cells. Our waste products and the breakdown of all living things, then enrich the soil with various compounds of nitrogen, which are recycled to make more protein.

CARBOHYDRATES

Carbohydrates are the chief source of energy in all living things. They contain carbon, hydrogen, and oxygen plus the sun's energy trapped in their combination.

There are various forms of carbohydrates. Sugars are the simplest, starches are more complex. All carbohydrate must be broken down into its simplest form of sugar before we can 'burn' it for energy. The process of breaking down starches into sugar takes place in the mouth, stomach and small intestines, through the presence of enzymes. These enzymes (ptyalin, amylase, and maltase primarily) break down carbohydrates into smaller and smaller units until they can be absorbed into the liver. In the liver the sugar is either converted into fat and stored, or is sent out to the cells in the form of glucose or stored as glycogen. In the presence of oxygen this 'fuel' can be burnt, giving off heat and energy.

Sugar

The pattern of sugar consumption in Britain has reached dangerous proportions in view of the link between excessive use of refined sugar and diabetes, arteriosclerosis, arthritis and

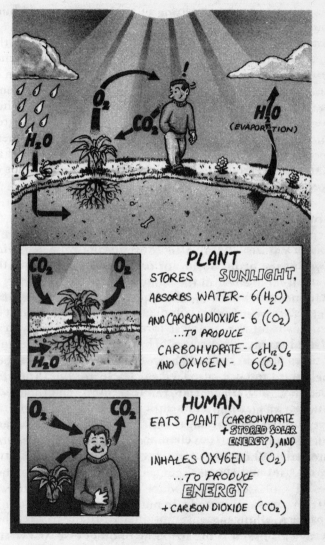

Figure 15

cancer, and it is not surprising to find that the incidence of these diseases is on the increase. In this century there has been an 80 per cent increase in coronary deaths and cancer in the UK. After all, our average daily refined sugar consumption is 130 pounds a year, 1000 per cent more than earlier this century. In fact, despite all our medical advances and increased expenditure on medicine and research, we still have the same life expectancy as 100 years ago. Changes in diet, and particularly refined sugar consumption, are at least partially responsible.

Yet if sugar is so destructive, why is it so attractive? Sugar in nature is contained mainly in fruit. The sweet part of the fruit usually surrounds the seed, and it is the sweetness that attracts man and animal to eat the fruit. By doing so the seed of the fruit is deposited on the earth, accompanied by some 'manure'. In this way nature uses man to continue the propagation and growth of the plant. Sugar not only provides us with energy, but the level of sugar in the blood controls our appetite. Our experience teaches us these things, and we develop a natural affinity for sweet foods.

Refined sugar

The problem started when we discovered that we could concentrate and refine natural sugars. Instead of eating fruit, we learnt how to concentrate the sweetness, and produced the substance we now know as sugar – pure, white and deadly. Like most foods in nature, sugar cane, the source of most sugar, comes equipped with the vitamins and minerals needed to use it properly. When sugar cane is refined all these nutrients are removed, leaving 100 per cent sucrose. By adding small quantities of molasses, a by-product of refining sugar, to white sugar, brown sugar is made. In nutritional terms it is not much different to white sugar.

Above all else, it is the stripping of other essential vitamins and minerals that render refined sugar so toxic. When glucose is burned in the cell to make energy, a cycle of reactions take place (known as the Krebs cycle) that require the presence of at least ten of these nutrients. Vitamins B_2, B_3, B_5, B_6, C and E and manganese, magnesium, chromium, calcium and zinc are the most important. If one of these nutrients is missing, the result could be an incompletely 'burned' compound being deposited in the cell. These compounds are very toxic, and with their build-up, physiological deterioration begins.

Blood sugar balance

Sugar also triggers the release of hormones from the adrenal glands and pancreas. Normally, these hormones function to raise our available energy. However, continued intake of sugar keeps our body in the state of 'red alert'. As time goes by the adrenals need even more sugar to produce the same energy reaction, so we increase our sugar intake to keep our energy up. Much like any addictive drug, we need more and more to get the same 'hit'.

Eventually our bodies can't handle so much sugar and the pancreas and adrenal glands stop producing enough hormones. Exhaustion, confusion, depression, diabetes, arthritis, infection and allergies are some of the symptoms of a long term overload of refined sugar.

Natural sugar

The most common form of natural sugar is fructose, found in fruit. Unlike glucose, fructose can enter into the cell and bloodstream without needing the release of insulin, a pancreatic enzyme. It is also absorbed more slowly and is therefore less likely to trigger a dramatic change in blood sugar level. If taken in the form of fruit it also contains the necessary vitamins and minerals.

Honey

For centuries honey has been renowned for its health-giving

properties, and through analysis of the ingredients in it we can begin to see why. The principal sugars in honey are levulose (or fructose) and dextrose, or glucose. The dextrose has an immediate effect on blood sugar, increasing available energy, while the levulose releases slowly into the blood, keeping the blood sugar level up for many hours after being gradually converted into glucose.

Unfortunately, most commercial honey is heated, to aid the processes of mixing different types of filtering, and the heat process turns a lot of these relatively harmless sugars into sucrose. There is also a destruction of enzymes and vitamins. For this reason it is important to use untreated honey which has not been heated above 114°F. This is usually available in good health food shops or from local beekeepers. Also, select the darker honeys as these contain more iron, copper and manganese and are less acidic.

Molasses

When sugar cane is processed to make sucrose, there are many by-products. Molasses is one of these by-products and contains a lesser proportion of sugar, plus minerals. Black strap molasses contains even less sugar and a significant quantity of iron, calcium, zinc, copper and chromium, which are needed to process the sugar.

Lactose

The sugar in milk is known as lactose, and is more complex in chemical structure than glucose or fructose. It requires a particular enzyme needed to break it down, called lactase. Milk, especially in non-fat, dried form, contains high protein, carbohydrate and substantial vitamin and mineral content. It has therefore been included in most overseas nutritional aid programmes. However, many aid recipients become ill from drinking this alien substance. Research into the cause, revealed that many cultures simply do not have the enzyme lactase and therefore cannot tolerate milk sugar. In the United States 70 per cent of the black population and 15 per cent of the white population are lactose intolerant. The symptoms are flatulence, bloating, abdominal cramps and sometimes diarrhoea.

Lactose intolerant people can still enjoy home made yogurt, buttermilk and cheese since the lactose in these foods is converted into lactic acid during the fermentation process. However, if a reaction still occurs with these foods there may be an allergy to some other constituent of milk.

Starches
Most carbohydrates in nature are in the form of starch, the major sources being seeds, grains, pulses and tubers such as potatoes. Starches can be thought of as complex sugars, requiring an even longer digestive process than milk sugar to break down to glucose. Thus, starches do not produce an immediate elevation of blood sugar.

Refined flours
At the beginning of this century we consumed twice as much starch as sugar. Now we consume more sugar than starch.

Like the sugar in fruit, most forms of starch come complete with the other nutrients needed to process them. If we refine these foods, stripping away the necessary vitamins and minerals, we end up poisoning ourselves with toxic by-products of incomplete metabolism.

Most wheat flour, like sugar, has been denutrientized through steel roller mills. As the grain is crushed the heat of the steel rollers destroys important vitamins. If that wasn't enough we also take out the bran and the germ, until we are left with almost pure starch. By removing these other ingredients it becomes possible to store white flour almost indefinitely without it 'going off'. At this stage it cannot even support the life of a weevil or a rat, yet we continue to feed it to ourselves. Another disadvantage of such refining is that it increases the proportion of gluten in the flour. Gluten is a sticky protein which is responsible for making bread springy. So in order to make a light loaf, high gluten flour is used. However, gluten binds B vitamins and sticks to the walls of the small intestine, decreasing absorption of vital nutrients.

Wholewheat stoneground flour

The best way to make wheat flour is to grind it between two stones and use the lot. Such wholewheat stoneground flour still contains valuable vitamins and minerals. However, as it can go rancid fairly quickly; do not buy a sack for many months' baking, buy a small amount at a time and keep it in a cool place.

While 100 per cent wholewheat bread made from stoneground flour is infinitely preferable to white bread or commercial 'brown' as opposed to wholewheat bread, it is wise to keep the intake of any wheat products down, because of the gluten content. There are many healthy alternatives: buckwheat, rice, corn, and soya flour will all add variety to your baking.

Whole grains

Of course, the least adulterated form of grain is wholegrain, simply boiled and eaten. This ensures the greatest intake of the vitamins and minerals contained within the grain. Crushing a grain for flour makes these vital nutrients become increasingly vulnerable.

A grain consists of three parts, the germ, the endosperm and the bran. The germ is the part which sprouts when the seed is planted, and is the most nutritious part of the grain. It contains large amounts of B vitamins and vitamin E, saturated oils, protein, carbohydrate and minerals. Once the germ, such as wheatgerm, has been separated from the grain, it can go rancid, so it should be kept in a cool place and eaten as soon as possible.

The endosperm is the largest part of the grain and consists

mainly of starch and protein. When flour is refined only the endosperm is left. The outer shell of a whole grain is bran: a largely indigestible carbohydrate complex rich in cellulose.

Cellulose

Cellulose acts as roughage in the diet and generally improves digestion. According to Dr Burkitt it also gives protection against diverticular disease, appendicitis, and cancer of the

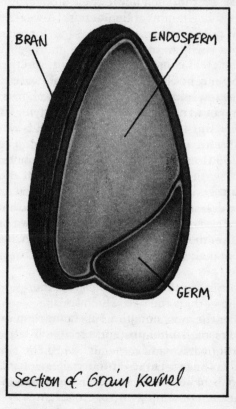

Section of Grain Kernel

Figure 16

colon. However, some plant foods, most notably grains, peas and beans, also contain a large proportion of phytic acid, which reacts with valuable minerals like calcium, iron and zinc and carries them out of the body. People who have become accustomed to a high fibre, and therefore high phytic acid, diet seem to have less trouble than those who have just changed their diet. But since there is little phytic acid and plenty of cellulose in raw vegetables, these are a better form of roughage than bran, at least for those changing their diet.

PROTEIN

Protein is the chief constituent of all cells, whether animal or vegetable. So our bodies consist largely of protein. It forms a structure around which calcium and phosphorus deposit to make bones. Hair and nails are made of protein. Collagen, the 'glue' between our cells, holding us together, is a protein. Our tendons, muscles and organs are made up of protein. Even enzymes, blood and many of our hormones contain protein.

Protein is synthesized within the plant with the aid of the sun, joining together carbon, oxygen, hydrogen and nitrogen (sometimes, also sulphur and phosphorus). Although 79 per cent of the air we breathe contains nitrogen, we cannot combine this with carbohydrates (made up of carbon, hydrogen and oxygen) to make protein. We can only use nitrogen trapped by plants.

Nitrogen cycle

Protein is a much more complex substance than carbohydrate and therefore each unit of protein is relatively large and heavy. A molecule of protein can be as much as 10,000 times as heavy as a molecule of sugar. These protein molecules are made up of a number of smaller units called amino acids. Amino acids ('amino' means containing nitrogen) eventually breakdown into ammonia which is nitrogen combined with hydrogen.

Ammonia and other waste products are then returned to the soil. Through the action of bacteria these nitrogen compounds are turned into nitrates, which are absorbed into the plant through its roots. The plant uses these nitrates to make more protein, and the cycle starts again.

A unit of protein consists of some 22 different amino acids. As we are able to make only 14 of these in our bodies, we must take in the remaining eight amino acids in our dietary protein. For this reason these eight are called essential amino acids. Not only do all eight have to be present in our food, but they must be present in the right proportions. If a food lacks one amino acid, then that food contains no usable protein.

A recent television advertisement for bread serves as a good illustration of this point. The advertisement stated that bread had more protein than an equivalent weight of cheese, milk or eggs. It then went on to say that protein is vital for our nutrition. Both these statements are true, but the assumption that bread

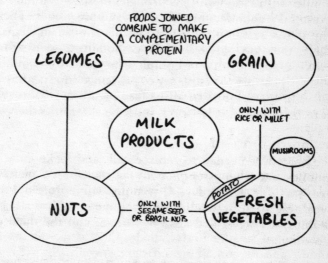

Figure 17

is therefore better for you than cheese, milk or eggs is not true – simply because bread lacks lysine. So bread has less usable protein than any of these foods. Similarly, while peanuts have more protein than an equivalent serving of meat, they contain less usable protein because they are low in the essential sulphur amino-acids.

Complete protein

Foods which contain all eight amino acids in approximately the right proportions are called complete proteins. The highest sources of complete protein are eggs, yogurt, raw milk, meat, fish and cheese. These foods eaten on their own provide us with usable protein. However, it is a mistake to think of these as our only sources of complete protein.

Complementary proteins

If one food has a deficiency in two amino acids, and it is combined with a food which is strong in these two amino acids, the result is a complete protein. For example, rice is deficient in the amino acids isoleucine and lysine, and broad beans are strong in these two amino acids. By combining these two foods, we have a good source of complete protein. By combining foods it is possible to get plenty of protein without eating any meat, fish, eggs or milk products (see Figure 18). Please note that to be effective these foods must be eaten together.

How much protein?

Since protein is needed to replace cells and make enzymes, hormones and other essential body substances, it is necessary to consume it every day. Optimum daily protein intake depends on three factors: life circumstances, individual needs and ability to digest and absorb protein, and the quality of the protein.

Life circumstances   Any situation in which your body is engaged

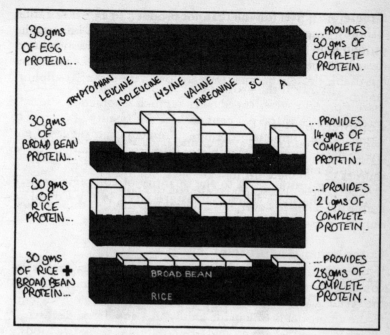

Figure 18

in building activities will increase your need for protein. For instance pregnant women, nursing mothers, or growing children need more protein. So do athletes and those recovering from operations or a long period without food. A manual worker will need more than someone sitting at a desk all day. In addition to this, any situation leading to the loss of nitrogen from your body will increase protein requirement. Excess sweating causes a slight loss of nitrogen and so do infections which decrease absorption through diarrhoea and increase excretion through excess urination.

Individual needs   Some of us require slightly more of one amino acid, and a few need more than the eight essential amino acids in their diet, because they cannot produce all 14 other amino acids. Absorption of protein is also dependent on enzyme production, and healthy intestines; the individual variation is considerable.

Protein quality   If the protein we eat contains only 50 per cent usable protein, we will need twice as much as someone who eats protein which is 100 per cent usable. The quality of protein is crucial. The complete protein requirement chart suggests sensible daily levels of complete protein. Remember, these amounts must not be compared to the quantity of food containing protein, but to the quantity of complete protein found in the food. These values are given in the Complete

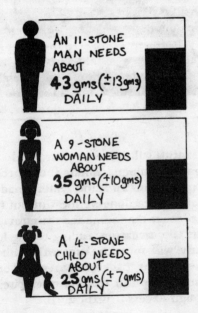

Figure 19

Protein chart. For example 100 g of yogurt contain 4 g of complete protein. So a pint of yogurt would give you more than half your daily protein requirement.

Protein for breakfast

When we digest protein, enzymes in the stomach and small intestine break it down into amino acids. Once these have been absorbed into the body, they are reconstructed into protein to carry out building jobs in the body. However, when dietary carbohydrate is short some amino acids will be converted into glucose in the liver and used as fuel rather than building materials. These converted amino acids give us a longer term supply of energy by releasing glucose slowly into the bloodstream, rather like starches.

By eating protein in the morning our blood sugar level stays at an even level for many hours. On the other hand coffee with sugar and toast will give us a sudden rise only to be followed by a sudden drop a couple of hours later. Then we reach for another hit of coffee or sugar. For this reason it is best to have half your daily protein needs in the morning, by eating yogurt, buttermilk or eggs.

Animal vs. vegetable

One of the most popular delusions about protein, is that it is impossible to get enough without eating meat. However, the majority of us could easily leave meat out of our diet and still get enough protein. In fact three-quarters of the world's population eat too much protein.

While it is true that meat contains a high proportion of good quality complete protein, there are many other factors that are not in its favour. Most importantly, in cooking our meat many essential vitamins are lost. Without them, meat can produce dangerous toxins. If we do not have adequate B_6 which is in raw meat but not cooked meat, one amino acid breaks down into a toxic substance related to arteriosclerosis. Indeed, in cultures eating a high proportion of meat, with the exception of Eskimos who eat it raw, there is a high rate of arteriosclerosis. Meat also contains excessive amounts of cholesterol and saturated fats which may contribute to its negative effect on the condition of our heart and arteries.

Certain parts of the animal are better than others. For instance, the liver contains vast quantities of vitamin A. Animals in the wild always eat the internal, nutritious organs first, leaving the tough supportive tissue (which we in the West prize most highly) to the last. Supportive tissue, the stuff a steak is made of, takes two days to digest completely. During this time the meat putrifies, destroying other nutrients and upsetting our correct balance of intestinal bacteria. Since the meat we eat is not quite as fresh as a lion's dinner, there is an even higher risk of putrefaction. Furthermore, our beef, pork, chicken and turkeys are usually treated with antibiotics, and other toxic drugs which store in the tissues and the liver. So if you eat meat, get free range chicken or lamb's liver.

Fish

Fish is a better form of protein than meat. It digests easily because it has a different type of supportive tissue, which, depending on the type of fish, for example, mackerel, is high in vitamin A and minerals and forms vitamin D as it breaks down. It is also a purer and cheaper form of protein than meat – cod and haddock are almost pure protein.

Eggs

As far as protein is concerned eggs are an excellent source. Their amino acid pattern closely matches our needs, so one egg will provide 6 g of complete protein. Most people believe them to be bad because they contain cholesterol, but they also contain lecithin. Provided our intake of lecithin matches our cholesterol intake there is little problem. However, lecithin is destroyed if you fry them or cook them in oil. So eat your eggs boiled or baked. About three eggs a week will cause no problems to blood cholesterol levels.

Dairy produce

Cottage cheese and yogurt are my favourite sources of protein. They are low in saturated fats and lactose (milk sugar), and high in protein, vitamins and minerals. Yogurt is delicious for breakfast with chopped banana, wheatgerm and ground sesame seeds.

Cheese and milk are also good sources of protein. However, milk does not agree with everyone (because of lactose intolerance and other allergies) and too much can cause excessive mucus production. Pasteurization also decreases the vitamin and mineral content. However, combining milk with grains, nuts, seeds, beans or potatoes considerably increases their complete protein content.

Vegetable protein

Soyabeans are the most complete form of vegetable protein – one-third of a cup of dried beans, cooked, gives you at least 10 g of complete protein. By combining this with grains, nuts or seeds the protein content will be further improved.

This is only one example of the many vegetable combinations that make complete proteins. It is time to drop the notion that we need meat to survive. Combined vegetables can easily cover our needs, as many vegetarians are aware. However, if you are a strict vegetarian (eating no meat, milk or eggs) it is hard to get enough B_{12}. While it is found in seaweed, yeast, wheatgerm, soyabeans and comfrey leaves, the quantities are low compared to dairy produce, eggs, and meat. If you have symptoms of tiredness, pallor, and a sore tongue or tingling hands or feet it is essential to take a B_{12} supplement. Vegans may also be deficient in zinc.

FATS

Animals and vegetables store energy in the form of fats and oils. When we eat fats, we can either use them for energy or store them as a reserve. Unlike starches, which are basically a combination of carbon and water (H_2O), fats are a combination of carbon and hydrogen with just a little oxygen. Each carbon atom can be attached to, at four places. Two of these are attached to adjacent carbon atoms, making a chain. Put simply, if the other two are attached to hydrogen atoms it is called saturated fat, because all available bonds have become saturated with hydrogen.

Saturated fats

Animals store their fat in saturated form, so the fat in meat and butter is saturated. One of the properties of saturated fat is solidity at room temperature. Also the longer the carbon chain, the more solid the fat will be. Butter has from 4 to 18 carbon links and melts easily, while beef fat has 14 to 18 carbon links, and is so solid it can be used to make candles. Fatty tissue surrounds our organs giving them protection, smoothing out our contours, as well as insulating and preserving heat. Fats also provide us with the fat soluble vitamins A, D, and E, and

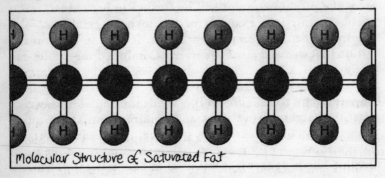

Molecular Structure of Saturated Fat

Figure 20

providing there is no lack of these, and no imbalance of the liver, gall-bladder or circulatory system, saturated fats are not harmful. However, if the lining of the arteries have started to form deposits, excess fatty acids in the blood can speed up the growth of these deposits. Also, fat which is not being burned as energy will result in weight gain, and will slow down our digestion considerably. It is thought that our liking for fats is connected with the lengthy time needed to digest them which gives us a sensation of being full.

Complete protein

Amount of complete protein in 100g of

Soya	20 g
Cheddar cheese	19 g
Beef, steak	17 g
Chicken	15 g
Fish, baked	14 g
Cottage cheese	13 g
Eggs (2)	12 g
Yogurt	4 g
Skimmed milk	3 g
Beans + rice	15 g
Beans + milk	15 g
Sesame + peanuts	11 g
Rice + sesame	5 g
Potato + milk	5 g

Unsaturated fats

When the loose bonds in the chain of carbon atoms are not 'saturated' with hydrogen, the fat is 'unsaturated'. Vegetables store their energy in the form of unsaturated and saturated fat. The more unsaturated the fat the more liquid it will be.

Cold pressed vegetable oils, like sesame, sunflower, soya and

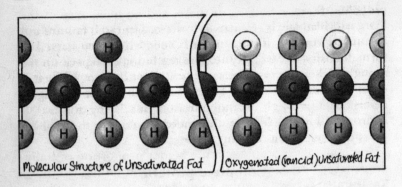

Molecular Structure of Unsaturated Fat | Oxygenated (rancid) Unsaturated Fat

Figure 21

safflower oil contain polyunsaturated fats which means that many (poly) of the bonds are free, while olive oil, which contains mono-unsaturated fats, has less free bonds.

Cold pressed oils must be refrigerated or eaten fresh otherwise they will gradually go rancid. Rancidity occurs when oxygen attaches itself to a free bond. This process happens very quickly when the oil is heated. The oxygen atoms can later detach themselves and latch onto another molecule such as a vitamin, destroying or damaging it. These dangerous oxygen based molecules are called free radicals, and can set up destructive chain reactions which damage cells, and can lead to excessive cell proliferation, causing arteriosclerosis. For this reason there is little advantage in cooking with cold pressed vegetable oils. They should be kept in the fridge and eaten with salads. It is best to avoid too many fried foods anyway. Vitamin E, since it is an anti-oxidant protects these oils from going rancid inside you. Most natural oils contain vitamin E, which helps to stabilize the oils. However, since there is no law about removing vitamin E from oils, some large oil companies remove the vitamin E, sell inferior oil, and then sell the vitamin E for supplementation to be taken by the people they helped make vitamin E deficient in the first place!

Margarine

Margarine is made by attaching hydrogen to the free bonds of an unsaturated fat. This process is called hydrogenation and turns the unsaturated fat into a saturated fat. The reason for doing this is to make it the same texture as butter. While it is technically a saturated fat, advertizing laws permit margarine labels to say 'high in polyunsaturates'. The process of hydrogenation not only saturates the fat, it changes the form and positions of the unsaturated bonds.

Some margarines do contain a higher proportion of unhydrogenated polyunsaturates, however, too much polyunsaturated fat is also not a good idea.

Essential fatty acids

Unsaturated oils contain three fatty acids which are known to be needed for normal growth, proper hormone balance and healthy blood, arteries and nerves. These are linoleic, alpha-linolenic and arachidonic acid, which used to be known collectively as vitamin F. Actually, arachidonic acid isn't essential in man because we can make it from linoleic acid. These essential fatty acids become more and more complex as they are processed by the body, and eventually turn into hormone-like substances called prostaglandins. These prostaglandins have numerous functions including reducing inflammation, controlling fats in the blood, and balancing sex hormones. Essential fatty acids and their derivatives also get incorporated into cell walls because fats provide the flexibility needed, for example, to make bendy, elastic arteries or smooth, elastic skin. They are also used to insulate nerves by surrounding the nerve with a myelin sheath.

In multiple sclerosis myelin shows signs of degeneration and this results in 'short circuits' causing a loss of muscle control. Multiple sclerosis sufferers have been shown to respond well to supplementation with essential fatty acids.

Linoleic acid is called a series 6 fatty acid because its first double bond occurs in the sixth place. Whatever the body does in processing this fat it always stays a series 6 fatty acid. The first step in the process converts it into gamma-linolenic acid, or GLA. GLA is found naturally in evening primrose oil, black-currant seeds, and the herb borage. Many people have difficulty turning the more abundant linoleic acid into GLA. This can be for genetic reasons or simply because of a diet too high in fat or alcohol, both of which make conversion less easy. Vitamin B_6, biotin, zinc, and magnesium are also needed to make GLA so deficiency of these nutrients can also cause GLA deficiency. GLA is then converted into another fatty acid and thence into prostaglandins series 1. These have an anti-inflammatory effect and help balance sex hormones. This is the likely reason why supplementation with evening primrose oil has been shown to help relieve eczema, asthma, allergic rhinitis, and PMT.

Alpha-linolenic acid, also rich in seeds, nuts, and vegetable oils, turns into EPA and from there into another fat called DHA. Prostaglandins series 3 are derived from EPA. These are all called n-3 or omega 3 fatty acids. EPA has been shown to have protective effects for the heart and arteries, keeping down fat and cholesterol levels, thinning the blood, and lowering blood pressure.

Balancing your fats

In the average Western diet, 42 per cent of calories are derived from fat. Above half of this is saturated fat (20 per cent of the total energy in the diet) and about a tenth is polyunsaturated (4.7 per cent of the total energy in the diet), the rest being monounsaturated fat. Current opinion is that the diet should obtain no more than 30 per cent of calories from fat, of which only about a third should come from saturated fat. In practical terms, this means eating less meat, eggs, dairy produce, and high fat convenience foods, and eating more vegetables, nuts and seeds, plus cold-pressed oils in salad dressings. Fish and chicken contain half the fat of beef and pork, and cottage cheese has about a third the fat of cheddar cheese.

Cholesterol

Another fat which has an essential role in the body is cholesterol. It is a normal component of body tissues, especially those of the brain, nervous system, liver and blood. It acts as a lubricant for the arteries, is needed to make adrenal and sex hormones, as well as vitamin D and bile, which digests fats.

Since gallstones and deposits found on the artery walls in arteriosclerosis contain cholesterol it has been theorized that they are caused by high cholesterol diets. But there is considerable evidence to show that the dietary intake of cholesterol need not be related to the body levels of cholesterol. It has been suggested that the cholesterol may even effect a 'puncture repair'. However, the build-up of cholesterol, fats, and calcium presents a later danger of arterial blockage. Excess cholesterol would therefore be a contributive factor, but not the only cause.

Lecithin

One substance which can break down cholesterol deposits, both in the arteries and gall-bladder (as in gallstones) is lecithin. It acts as a washing up liquid in that it breaks down fats into tiny particles that can be carried through the walls of the arteries and out of the blood. Bile, the digestive secretion from the gall-bladder, contains lecithin which breaks down fats into smaller units which the pancreas enzyme lipase can then work on.

Lecithin is found in soyabeans and corn; lecithin supplements usually being extracted from soyabeans.

SUN, SALT AND WATER

Sun

One thing we all take for granted is that the sun will rise every morning. It is absolutely fundamental to life and to nutrition. It is so fundamental that we often forget it is our primary source of energy. Not only does the sun provide us with heat and light, its energy is also trapped in the making of plant protein, carbohydrate and fat. Carbohydrate is made from the components carbon, hydrogen and oxygen. But if you were to get a measure of each and put them together nothing would happen. You'd still be left with carbon, hydrogen and oxygen. Yet in the presence of sunlight, the plant can combine these three ingredients, making much more than the sum of the components. The energy of the sun that is trapped in the plant is released in us when we eat it.

If we follow this principle through it would seem logical that some foods would have more sun energy, or vitality, than others. For instance, a freshly picked apple has more vitality than a slice of bacon. One possible way of quantifying this vitality is to add up the number of changes the food has been through since its 'birth'. An apple is in its original form and can be called 'first class vitality'. A slice of bacon may be the result of cooking a pig, that was fed cooked meat leftovers, that came from a cow that ate grass. The original form of grass is eaten by a cow. If we eat a cow raw it has 'second class vitality'. If we cook the cow it has 'third class vitality'. We then feed it to a pig, making 'fourth class vitality' food, and cook the pig, arriving at 'fifth class vitality' food. So in terms of vitality bacon doesn't come out very well.

First class vitality foods are raw fruits and vegetables, while second class vitality foods are cooked fruit, vegetables, grains and pulses, or herbivorous animal produce such as milk, raw eggs, cheese or raw steak. A cooked steak would have third class vitality, (see Figure 22).

This method of analysing foods is just a theoretical way of quantifying the life energy which is so obviously present in food, yet seems to elude scientific measurement. It has no relation to the specific protein or vitamin content in the food, which are also important to food value.

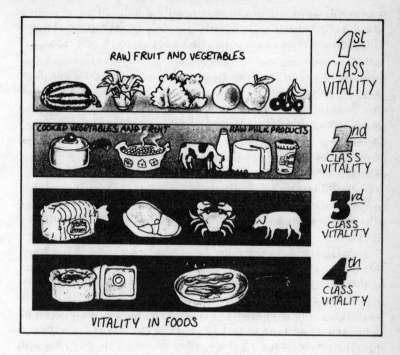

RAW FRUIT AND VEGETABLES — 1st CLASS VITALITY

COOKED VEGETABLES AND FRUIT — RAW MILK PRODUCTS — 2nd CLASS VITALITY

3rd CLASS VITALITY

4th CLASS VITALITY

VITALITY IN FOODS

Figure 22

Water

Like the sun, water is a basic necessity of life. A lack of it prevents our body from flourishing, causes our health to deteriorate and the ageing process to accelerate. Most of us suffer from insuffient water, and 'dry out' as the years go by. A dry skin, cracked lips and stiff joints are some of the outward signs of a lack of water, yet we usually attribute these obvious signs of dehydration and a lack of lubrication to some other cause.

Our bodies consist of 65 per cent water, contained in every single cell. Without water cells cannot function, nor can we digest and eliminate our foods so easily. Plenty of water flushes the digestive system and usually stops constipation. It also dilutes the urine, decreasing the concentration of toxins and the possibility of urinary infections.

To keep our body fluids balanced, we need about four pints of water every day. The need will, of course, vary with each individual. A diet high in fruit and salad may provide one and a half to two pints of water, and other beverages in the day may provide a pint. So, when your diet is good you will still benefit from at least a pint of water a day. If you drink tea, coffee, cocoa, alcohol or use diuretic drugs or salt your need for water will be higher.

While drinking a pint or two of water a day may sound like an effort, it has to be the cheapest way of cleansing the body and keeping healthy – even if it's bottled spring water!

Salt

Our bodies need the correct balance between sodium (salt) and potassium. Many years ago, before salt began to be used to flavour and preserve foods, our diets were predominantly high in potassium and low in salt. In order to maintain the elemental equilibrium we would have needed to retain most of the salt and excrete the excess potassium.

Our diets are now higher in salt than potassium, a complete reversal of our ancestors' diet, and we do not seem to have adapted physiologically to this change. While salt is not in itself bad, in excess it acts as an adrenal stimulant and encourages hypertension, arteriosclerosis and the retention of water in the fatty tissue (cellulite). It also damages the kidneys, upsets hormonal balance and is mildly addictive.

If you would have difficulty giving up the use of salt on foods and in cooking, the chances are your salt intake is too high. There is plenty of salt found naturally in foods, so there is no need to add extra. After two weeks without it your sense of taste is accentuated and the addition of salt seems unnecessary.

ACID AND ALKALINE

Our health depends upon the right balance of acid and alkaline within the body. The stomach must be acid to digest protein. The small intestines must be alkaline for their digestive processes to work, likewise the blood must be balanced 80 per cent alkaline 20 per cent acid.

To balance our bodies we must balance our diet with 80 per cent alkaline forming foods and 20 per cent acid forming foods. This is not simply the pH value of a food, it is the pH value of the 'ash' of the food once it has been 'burned' or metabolized. So oranges, which have a pH acid, are alkaline forming because they leave an alkaline ash in the body.

Normally the body keeps reserves of alkalines which can be used to neutralize excess acidity. However, an excess of acid forming foods will deplete reserves. Over-acidity is a cause of rheumatism, arthritic conditions and other diseases. Bacon and eggs, toast and coffee is an all acid way to start the day.

The effect of eating 80 per cent alkaline 20 per cent acid forming foods goes beyond simply improving health and resistance. It also affects our attitudes and feelings. Over acidity tends to bring out our aggression and negativity, and a sense of life being a great effort. While balancing 80/20 brings out positive feelings, and a sense of continuity or flow in life, in which there is no need for stress. Acidity provides a grounding influence, while alkalinity is more enlightening and enlivening.

COMBINING FOODS

Since different foods require different enzymes to digest them, indigestion can result from combining the wrong foods. The most common symptom of wrongly combined foods is sleepiness after meals, indigestion and bloatedness. Under normal conditions careful food combining is not essential, as our bodies are amazingly adaptive. However, if you have digestive

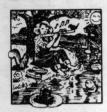

BALANCE
80% Alkaline

Vegetables			
soya beans	4	lemon	2
lima beans	4	nectarine	2
spinach	4	orange	2
turnips	4	gooseberries	2
beetroot and tops	4	raspberries	2
kelp	4	strawberries	2
carrots	3	grapefruit	1
celery	2	tomato	1
cucumber	2	peach	1
lettuce	2	melon	1
parsley	2	cherries	1
parsnips	2	apples	1
radish	2	grapes	1
watercress	2	pears	1
potatoes	2	bananas	1
runner beans	2	watermelon	1
cauliflower	2	prunes	1
dandelion greens	2	**Proteins**	
cabbage	1	almonds	3
asparagus	1	millet	1
leeks	1	brazil nuts	1
marrow	1	coconuts	1
onions	1	buckwheat	1
		Other	
Fruits		herb teas	2
figs	4		
apricots	4	**Neutral Foods**	
raisins	3	vegetable oils	
dates	3	white sugar	
pineapple	2	butter	
currants	2	raw milk	
blackberries	2		

YOUR DIET
20% Acid

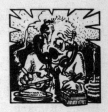

Vegetables	
lentils	1
peas	1
beans, dried	1

Fruits	
rhubarb	1
canned, sugared, glazed or preserved fruits	1

Proteins	
oysters	4
lobsters	4
veal	4
fish	3
eggs	3
organ meats	3
chicken	3

most meats and fowl	3
most grains	3
rice	2
wholewheat/rye bread	2
nuts other than almonds and brazils	2
mutton	2
beef	2
cheese	1
boiled, pasteurized milk	1
peanuts	1

Acidic drinks
tea
coffee
cocoa
chocolate

Key: 1 = mildly acid/alkaline forming
2 = medium acid/alkaline forming
3 = strongly acid/alkaline forming
4 = very strongly acid/alkaline forming

difficulties, it is wise to check how sensitive you are to certain food combinations.

Protein and starch

Protein requires the presence of hydrochloric acid in the stomach to be digested, and starch does not as it is not digested in the stomach. The combining of a concentrated protein, such as an egg, with a concentrated starch, such as potato, often results in indigestion. However, by eating the protein first and then the starch, the stomach can stack these foods in layers. Since hydrochloric acid is more concentrated in the bottom half of the stomach, the food will be digested more easily if eaten this way.

Fruit

Unlike most other foods, fruit usually passes through the stomach in 90 minutes. If it is eaten with any other food it may stay in the stomach too long and start to ferment, so it is better to eat it between meals and leave an hour after a meal before having some fruit.

Yogurt

Fruit, with the exception of banana, does not combine well with yogurt. The different digestive processes in the stomach partially destroy the beneficial effect the yogurt bacteria normally have on the intestines. Also the taking of vitamin C at the same time as yogurt has been reported to decrease the absorption of this valuable vitamin.

Drinking

While water, juices and herb teas are health promoting, drinking during a meal will dilute the digestive juices. Since different foods contain different amounts of water it is hard to say exactly how much one may drink during a meal. Basically, it is better to restrict oneself to a small glass of water, or wine, which can aid digestion.

FASTING

Fasting comes naturally to animals and children when they are sick, yet for so many people, the thought of a few days without food often seems like a threat to survival itself! Fasting not only cleanses the body, bringing increased vitality, but it also breaks the habit of eating, allowing us a new perspective to the role of food in our lives.

By abstaining from food, the body begins to release stored toxins into the blood, for elimination through the kidneys. This elimination process is most active during the first day and often causes slight headaches and nausea. By drinking plenty of liquid and taking 100mg of niacin, 2g of vitamin C and 50mg of potassium twice a day, the body detoxifies more effectively, the kidneys are well supported, and the 'symptoms' are less uncomfortable. Niacin in the form of nicotinic acid flushes out toxins from the capillaries and brings on a blushing sensation for 15 to 30 minutes. Vitamin C detoxifies poisons being released into the bloodstream, and potassium supports the kidneys, and helps to release excess salt from the body. The best fluids to drink are spring water with fresh lemon juice, or diluted sugar-free grape juice. Make sure you drink at least 3 pints (1½ litres) a day.

Once the body has thrown off toxins and burnt all available glucose, it begins to break down fatty tissue to be used as energy. As the fat is burned, toxic by-products will be produced if there is not an adequate supply of the vitamins and minerals needed during the process of oxidation. To ensure an adequate supply it is best to precede a fast by at least one week of extremely nutritious eating, and take a high strength B complex during the fast.

Fasting is not recommended for people with the symptoms of a lack of nutrients, or an inability to use these nutrients, since a fast would simply increase the deficiency. For such people, a build-up period of maybe a month is recommended before starting a 3 to 5 day fast.

A gentler and effective method of cleansing the body is to eat only grapes, and drink plenty of grape juice and water for the 3 to 5 days. Grapes are extremely alkaline and contain plenty of minerals, especially potassium.

HOW GOOD IS YOUR DIET?

Most of the time, eating is a habitual automatic exercise. While the act of eating is best left habitual (otherwise death ensues), what you eat and when you eat it is often ingrained from our childhood, and what our parents and schools taught us. Some of these habits may be good, but some of them may not support your health at all. In order to be able to consciously choose the habits you would like to keep, your attachment to habitual eating will have to change.

Breaking the habits

Ask yourself honestly which foods and drinks you would find most difficult to give up. The most common habitual foods are bread, milk, cheese, tea and coffee. Not surprisingly, they are also the most common allergens (foods to which people develop an allergy), which arise because the body can no longer cope with the continuous digestion of one food type. Only when you can go without your 'staple foods' for a month, without craving them, can you begin to choose which foods suit you best.

For myself, I found that giving up milk and wheat was almost impossible. However, after a month I felt so much better that I now eat a smaller quantity of these foods, which I can tolerate and enjoy without any adverse effects.

How healthy is your diet?

The following questions may help you to decide which areas of your diet you would most like to change.

Your diet

How many tablespoons of sugar do you eat in one day?

Do you use salt in your cooking?

Do you add salt to your food?

How many coffees do you have a day?

How many teas?

How many cigarettes do you smoke each day?

Do you take any other non-medical drugs?
(i.e. cannabis, amphetamines, etc.)

What is your usual alcoholic drink?

How many do you have a week?

How many times a week do you have fried food meals?

How many times a week do you have red meat?
(beef, pork, lamb, game)

How many times a week do you have white meat?
(poultry, fish)

How many times a week do you eat pasta or pastry?

How much milk do you drink a week?

Do you eat yogurt?

Do you go out of your way to avoid foods with additives or preservatives?

How many slices of bread do you eat each week?

Do you eat chocolate more than twice a week?

How much plain water do you drink a day?

What percentage of your diet is raw fruit and raw vegetables?

What food or drinks would you have difficulty giving up?

Write down all foods and drinks consumed in the last three days, listing them as follows, so that you can see your habitual eating patterns.

	Day 1	Day 2	Day 3
Breakfast			
Lunch			
Dinner			

The next section will help you choose a healthier diet.

BUILDING A BETTER DIET

While there are principles of nutrition that apply to us all, we are individuals and our needs are unique. Therefore there is no one right answer to the questions in the previous section. You must experiment with your diet, be creative and learn from your experiences. Above all, enjoy what you eat.

Here are some simple guidlines and recipes to help you get started. Change your diet at your own pace, and don't feel guilty when you eat something 'bad' – chocolate eaten guiltily is twice as harmful! Just notice the effects of the foods you eat and choose the ones that make you feel good.

1 Get plenty of exercise and fresh air.
2 Make sure you are getting enough (not too much) complete protein, preferably in the first half of your day.
3 Use cold pressed oils for salads, and eat few fried foods.
4 Avoid sugar, salt, coffee and other adrenal stimulants.
5 Eat whole grains and avoid foods containing preservatives and additives.
6 Eat plenty of raw vegetables, helping to keep three-quarters of your diet alkaline forming food.
7 Decrease meat consumption, fish and free range chicken being preferable.
8 Eat plenty of raw fruit between meals.
9 Drink a pint of water a day between meals.
10 Keep your intake of bread, pasta and pastry low.
11 Eat when you are relaxed and hungry.
12 Do not overeat.

Diet for whole health

On rising Herb tea or spring water	*Gives you*
Breakfast 10 oz (285g) plain yogurt with banana, wheatgerm, sunflower and sesame seeds, and bran/scrambled eggs/muesli.	Complete protein, plenty of vitamins and minerals, and yogurt for alkalinity and bacterial health.

Mid morning

Fruit, water, fruit juice, herb tea or dandelion coffee.

Vitamin C, some minerals and plenty of fibre.

Lunch

Salad – a selection of the following: lettuce, celery, cucumber, carrot (including tops), raw beetroot or parsnip, cress, watercress, chinese leaves, leek, onion, pepper, parsley, with dressing, and vegetable quiche/ egg mayonnaise/cheese/fish/ vegetable pies or stews.

More protein, starch and plenty of fibre. Vitamins and minerals in vegetables, essential fatty acids in salad dressing, correct acid/alkaline balance.

Mid afternoon

Fruit salad/dried fruit, and herb tea of Rooibosch tea.

Vitamin C, some minerals and plenty of fibre.

Dinner

Leek/lentil soup, salad as for lunch, stir fried vegetables, vegetable stew/baked potatoes/glass of wine.

Easily digested carbohydrate with some roughage. Alkaline.

Before bed

Herb tea/spring water.

3

VITAMINS AND MINERALS

At the beginning of this century a chain of discoveries were made, which could have changed the entire course of medicine, had we been ready for it. These were the discoveries of vitamins A, B and C.

Unlike protein, fat or carbohydrates, vitamins are not used for energy or building materials. Yet without them there can be no energy and no cells. In a sense they are the nuts and bolts that hold us together. They are catalysts, they are regulators and most of all they are essential for life itself.

Vitamins are made in the green leaves of plants and are transferred into the seed of the plant to nourish the next generation. As we cannot make most vitamins, we rely on plants, and animals that have eaten the plants, to obtain sufficient quantities of these nutrients.

In the last 70 years we have isolated some twenty vitamins, which are classified into two groups. The fat soluble vitamins are vitamins A, D, E, F and K, and the water soluble vitamins include vitamins B, C and P. To maintain and promote health all these vitamins must be present in our diets in the right amounts.

In the sections that follow two levels of vitamin dosage are given. The RDA, 'recommended daily amount', is calculated as the average amount required, representing the requirements of 97 per cent of a population. People may be at risk of actual deficiency symptoms if they regularly consume less than 70 per cent of RDA. The 'optimum level' provides a range of supplementation, based on controlled research under medical supervision, that is safe and effective. These doses are not prescriptive. It is up to the reader to find the levels that suit them best, as individual variation is considerable.

It is possible that some individuals may suffer allergic reactions from the use of various dietary supplements or the media in which they are contained; if such reactions occur, consult your doctor. The author and publisher assume no responsibility.

WHY TAKE SUPPLEMENTS?

The predominant view held by the medical profession regarding vitamins is well summed up in 'Looking After Yourself', a booklet produced by the Health Education Council. It says 'if you're eating a fairly varied diet it is just about impossible to go short of proteins, vitamins or minerals. Vitamin pills aren't likely to help and as for minerals there is no shortage in the average British diet. As far as these nutrients are concerned we've never had it so good.'

How common is deficiency?

The Department of Health established recommended daily amounts (RDA) of vitamins which should be supplied in the diet to prevent deficiency. In 1980 a nationwide survey revealed the diet of 85 per cent of the British population to be deficient in at least one of these vitamins. In 1986, the Booker Health report backed up these findings in a survey which showed that 62 per cent of women and 45 per cent of men had less than the RDA for vitamin A; the average intake of vitamin E was only half the US RDA (there isn't any RDA in Britain); and that over 90 per cent of people got less than 2mg of B_6 a day, the US RDA. It also found that 60 per cent of women of reproductive age had iron intakes below the RDA and that

57 per cent of all women got less than 15mg of zinc, the US RDA. Clearly the average diet, even if it is fairly varied, does not cover most people's minimum nutritional requirements. If we look at the changing pattern of food consumption we can begin to see why.

Since the 1940s the consumption of fruit and vegetables, both high in vitamins, has dropped by 25 per cent, while the consumption of junk foods, lacking in nutrients, is up some 80 per cent. This increase in junk foods which consist largely of fat and sugar, also increases our need for vitamins. Pollution, many medical drugs, and food additives, all of which are on the increase, further tend to make us vitamin deficient, and so amplify our need for vitamin supplements.

Furthermore, the food we eat that does contain vitamins has less than it did thirty years ago. Why? Because our soil is increasingly being depleted of its essential nutrients, by over farming and because toxic insecticides kill off the micro-organisms that naturally revitalize the soil. In addition the processing of food usually substantially reduces its vitamin content.

Optimum nutrition not deficient nutrition

Perhaps the greatest misconception about vitamins is the notion that we only need them in small amounts, to correct deficiency. Firstly, the idea that the lack of a nutrient merely causes a deficiency disease is incorrect. Each vitamin has so many parts to play that any vitamin deficiency will disrupt our entire health. For instance, vitamin C keeps our arteries healthy, protects us from infections, takes poisons out of the body, and is involved in the production of energy. If we have insufficient vitamin C our heart and arteries deteriorate, our immune system is weakened, and production of energy is disrupted long before the advent of scurvy, the 'vitamin C deficiency' disease. It is time we started to think about the levels of vitamins that will promote optimum health, and not the levels that will prevent illness. The concept of a vitamin to cure a disease, is simply a variation of a 'drug to kill a bug'. The question we should be asking is how did the bug or disease get there in the first place? If improper nutrition was a causative factor, then how can that person improve his nutrition? By approaching the cause of disease there is no need to treat the symptoms. They will just clear up as part of the healing process.

Your needs are individual

There are situations when our need for vitamins is in excess of RDA levels. Our needs are higher when:

1   We are recovering from an illness
2   We are correcting a deficiency
3   A deficiency has caused a permanently increased need for a vitamin
4   We are stressed or engaged in extreme physical work
5   We are exposed to pollutants, medical drugs, toxic foods and food additives which rob us of nutrients.

Basically, almost all of us can benefit from taking supplements, and the amount to take will depend on your individual needs.

FAT SOLUBLE VITAMINS

The fat soluble vitamins are A, D, E, F and K. They are supplied to us in fats and oils, which are then absorbed in the digestive tract first into the lymphatic vessels and then into the blood for transport around the body. They can be stored in the body, so they do not need to be supplied on a daily basis. They are usually measured in International Units or IUs, which is a quality based measurement. For example, 13,500mcg of beta carotene, the vegetable form of vitamin A, is equivalent in potency to 750mcg of vitamin A oil, from fish liver. Both equal 2500 IU of vitamin A. The standards against which IUs are set are as follows:

1 IU of vitamin E = 0.67mg of d alpha tocopherol (E)
1 IU of vitamin A = 0.60mcg of beta carotene (A)
1 IU of vitamin D = 0.025mcg of pure vitamin (D)

Vitamin A

Vitamin A is mainly supplied as beta carotene, a reddish yellow substance found in foods such as carrots, beet, spinach, kale, broccoli and apricots. However, a much more usable form of this vitamin is found in liver and kidneys. Most vitamin A capsules contain fish liver oil.

What does it do?   The fact that liver, high in this vitamin, can prevent night blindness was known to the Egyptians many thousands of years ago. What they didn't know was that it strengthens against infection, improves the condition of the skin, both inside (the digestive tract and mucous membranes) and outside. It also slows down signs of ageing, helps prevent cancer, and is needed to make protein and sex hormones.

Vitamin A strengthens the outside surfaces of our body. Sufficient quantity means less spots and dryness of the skin. It protects our 'inside' skin against ulcers and viral invasions of the digestive tract, which cause diarrhoea and gastrointestinal disorders. It also protects our lungs and has been successfully used in the treatment of bronchitis.

Many of the so-called ageing symptoms, such as loss of smell, worsening eye sight and hearing, may be the result of a deficiency of this essential nutrient. With the discovery of RNA and its role in slowing down the ageing process, it has also been discovered that RNA production is proportional to the amount of vitamin A in the liver. So, the more vitamin A we have, the less we age. As RNA is also needed to make body protein it is not surprising to find that we can use dietary protein much better if we have adequate levels of vitamin A.

How much do you need Your need for vitamin A goes up if you eat too much protein, breathe polluted air, or are recovering from an infection. Since research by BUPA recently showed that a low or non existent level of vitamin A was found in the blood of people who subsequently got cancer, it is wise to get plenty of this vitamin.

   Deficiency symptoms are night blindness, ulcers, infections, loss of hearing and smell, dry skin, slow healing of cuts, loss of appetite and diarrhoea.

RDA: 2500 IU   Optimum level: 10,000–50,000 IU
Toxic level: 200,000 IU for prolonged length of time, although toxicity has occurred at 5000 IU regular intake.

Vitamin D

Vitamin D can be made in the skin in the presence of sunshine. However, since Britain cannot boast of hot summers, it is necessary to get the bulk of it from your diet. The major sources are milk, liver and egg yolk.

What does it do?   Vitamin D is necessary for healthy thyroid and parathyroid function by helping regulate the absorption and distribution of calcium. For this reason it is essential for healthy bones and teeth. Perhaps the lack of sunshine accounts for Britain's extraordinarily high incidence of rheumatism and arthritis.

   Deficiency symptoms are rickets, pyorrhoea, osteoporosis, retarded growth, weakness and lack of vigour.

How much do you need?   The amount you need depends on your exposure to sunlight, so in winter your need will be greatest.

RDA: 400 IU for children and housebound adults. For others 100 IU. Optimum level: 400–4000 IU
Toxic level: 100,000 IU

Vitamin E

There are many forms of this vitamin, called alpha, beta, gamma and delta tocopherol and so on. However, the most effective is alpha tocopherol. It is an oil and is found in many sources, the richest of which are green leafy vegetables, whole grains and especially wheatgerm. The oil of wheatgerm is most commonly used for vitamin E supplements.

What does it do? Perhaps its greatest asset, like vitamin C, is that it protects other substances in the body from oxidizing. It stops the destruction of unsaturated fats, hormones and other vitamins, and by sacrificing itself to these toxic oxides, it leaves the red blood cells supplied with pure oxygen, improving the functioning of the muscles. It also allows the cells to function with less oxygen. For these reasons it is excellent for many heart conditions, and situations in which there is restriction of blood flow. After its due publicity last decade, an estimated 35 million Americans were taking therapeutic levels of vitamin E. For the first time in medical history there was actually a decrease, not the normal rise, in the number of deaths from heart attacks.

This vitamin also acts as an anti-coagulant, being good for thrombosis, and is excellent for healing scars. It keeps our cells younger and therefore retards the ageing process, also promoting beautiful skin.

How much do you need? Inorganic iron, oestrogen, and unsaturated oils put up your need for vitamin E. So if you take the Pill you will need more vitamin E and if you take iron supplements containing ferric not ferrous iron, leave ten hours before taking vitamin E. The dietary sources of vitamin E are not commonly eaten in sufficient quantities to supply more than 15 IUs, so some nutritionists recommend supplementing this vitamin. People with high blood pressure should not take more than 100 IUs to start with, increasing the dose by 100 IUs each month. Chronic rheumatic heart disease patients should only receive vitamin E under medical supervision.

RDA: Not established   Optimum level: 400–2000 IU
Toxic level: Not established

Vitamin F

Vitamin F consists of the essential unsaturated fatty acids, linoleic, linolenic and arachidonic acid. It is found in the germ of grains, and in the seeds, and is therefore in vegetable oil.

What does it do?   Like other nutrients, certain types of fat are of vital importance. They are used as part of the structure of every cell, must be present for healthy nerves and brain, and help make adrenal, thyroid and sex hormones. Of these essential fats, only those constituting vitamin F cannot be made within us and must be obtained from our diet. These fats also nourish the skin and help to regulate blood coagulation, and can dissolve cholesterol deposits on artery walls. For this reason vitamin F is good for arteriosclerosis and heart disease.

Some people, especially those with multiple sclerosis, cannot transfer these fatty acids into gamma-linolenic acid, which is the form the body can use. Luckily for these people the oil of evening primrose contains vitamin F as gamma and linolenic acid.

How much do you need?   The need for vitamin F increases in proportion to the amount of saturated fat eaten. Saturated fat should only make up a third of all fat intake, the rest being cold pressed vegetable oils. As these are the source of vitamin F there is no need to supplement one's diet provided it contains at least 4 tablespoonsful of these oils.

RDA: Not established   Optimum level: 5 tablespoonsful
Toxic level: None known

Vitamin K

Vitamin K is a valuable part of your body's first aid kit. Without it you would bleed to death when you cut yourself, as it is essential for blood clotting. You can manufacture your own vitamin K, provided the right bacteria, promoted by eating yoghurt, are present in the intestines, otherwise it must be obtained from green vegetables, kelp, carrots, tomatoes and potatoes.

What does it do? Apart from clotting blood, it helps in the process of storing energy (glycogen) in the cells. It is also thought to be a factor in promoting vitality and long life.

How much do you need? It is very rare to have a deficiency of this vitamin unless there is a restriction of fat absorption. Antibiotics will decrease its availability by destroying intestinal bacteria, and a lot more of this vitamin may be used to stop prolonged menstruation.

Optimum level: An intake of 500 mcg, which is easily supplied in our diet, is sufficient for good health.

WATER SOLUBLE VITAMINS

Vitamin B complex and C are water soluble vitamins. They are present in vegetables, fruit, seeds and animal products. We absorb them through the digestive tract, from where they are taken to the liver, and transported around the body in the blood. Any unused B or C vitamin is readily excreted from the body so it is important to ingest them on a daily basis. They are usually measured in grams, milligrams (one thousandth of a gram) or micrograms (one millionth of a gram).

B Complex

Some fourteen separate vitamins make up the B complex and no doubt more will be added to this list as time goes on. While individual B vitamins have specific functions, they are supplied together in nature and work together in our bodies. They help determine our moods and mental attitude, promote healthy blood and circulation, improve our vitality and ability to cope with stress, keeping us young and energetic. The highest dietary sources are yeast, wheatgerm, whole grains, seeds, nuts, black strap molasses, green vegetables, legumes, milk products, liver and eggs.

B₁ Thiamine

Since thiamine is needed for burning glucose in the cell, and for making the important nerve chemical acetylcholine, it is not surprising to find beri-beri, a disease of the nervous system, as one of its deficiency symptoms. Thiamine also aids protein metabolism, the muscle tone of the digestive system, promoting growth, good appetite and the healthy functioning of the digestive tract. Deficiency of thiamine will therefore affect digestion, growth processes, energy production and, most of all, the brain and nervous system.

How much do you need? Deficiency symptoms occur among those who eat refined grains, most notably polished rice, and few raw vegetables. Like most B vitamins, thiamine is destroyed by heat and is contained in the germ of grains. Alcohol metabolism also uses up excessive amounts of B_1; so alcoholics are usually deficient.

RDA: 1.2mg   Optimum level: 25–250mg
Toxic level: None known

B₂ Riboflavin

Riboflavin is an orange yellow fluorescent chemical found in small amounts in vegetables, meat, milk, yeast and wheatgerm. It is essential for manufacturing the enzymes used to metabolize fats, proteins and carbohydrates. It is also needed for normal growth and tissue maintenance, and helps to neutralize acidity created when nutrients are burned to make energy.

The deficiency symptoms such as bloodshot, itchy eyes, sore tongue, dull oily hair, eczema, cataracts, cracked lips and mouth are all signs of over acidity.

How much do you need? Unlike other vitamins, riboflavin is primarily destroyed by light, so milk is not such a reliable source.

RDA: 1.6mg   Optimum level: 25–250mg
Toxic level: None known

B₃ Niacin (nicotinic acid or nicotinamide)

This nutrient comes in two forms, each with two different names. Nicotinic acid, is different from niacinamide, or nicotinamide, in that a sufficient dose of the former will cause vasodilation, which is characterized by a blushing and slightly itchy sensation. This effect is good and is used to improve circulation and detoxify the capillaries. It is therefore recommended during a fast. Niacin is intimately involved in metabolism and the burning of sugars to form energy, the regulation of blood sugar levels and histamine, and helps to keep down blood cholesterol. Because of its many roles it is useful in treating arteriosclerosis, arthritis, acne, depression, hypoglycaemia, alcoholism, headaches, and of course pellagra, for which it was discovered. It has been used in large amounts to successfully treat schizophrenia. Its overall character is one of expansion, releasing emotional and physiological blocks, and grounding. Perhaps its role in schizophrenia, and moments of high stress or tension is in bringing the person back to reality and grounding them.

How much do you need? It is needed in much larger quantities than most B vitamins, and since it is involved in sugar and carbohydrate metabolism even more must be supplied to those who eat plenty of sugars and starches. The individual variation in the need for this vitamin can be enormous. Flushing occurs with doses in excess of 100mg of nicotinic acid and usually lasts for 15 minutes.

RDA: 18mg   Optimum level: 50–500mg
Toxic level: 3,000–10,000mg

B_5 Pantothenic acid

Pantothenic acid is in almost all foods, hence its name, pantos meaning everywhere. This is just as well, because the number of roles B_5 plays in our bodies is enormous. It is needed for energy production, fat and cholesterol synthesis, antibody formation, manufacture of nerve chemicals, and, most of all, it is needed for the adrenal glands. By strengthening the adrenal glands and improving the production of cortisone, B_5 increases your resistance to stress. As a result of its anti-stress quality, it has been found very useful in treating rheumatism and arthritis.

How much do you need?   The deficiency symptoms like fatigue, desire to sleep a lot, loss of appetite, constipation, discontent and irritability, and lowered resistance to infections are very common. Yet few people are aware of this vitamin's importance.

RDA: Not established   Optimum level: 50–1000mg
Toxic level: None known

B_6 Pyridoxine

B_6 has so many functions it is hard to know where to start! It makes hormones, enzymes, nerve chemicals. It is needed for protein, carbohydrate, and fat metabolism. It makes antibodies, is needed to absorb B_{12}, and helps regulate sodium/potassium balance. 100mg a day for a couple of months will stop the symptoms of premenstrual syndrome in some people. It can relieve morning sickness, post natal depression, nervousness, hormone imbalances, kidney stones and digestive difficulties. Its essential role in making pancreatic enzymes also makes it vital for allergics and diabetics. It is also a natural analgesic and can be used to relieve pain. It is often wise to give it with zinc since these two nutrients work together.

How much do you need?   So many processes rob food of B_6, including cooking. But probably the most damaging of all is

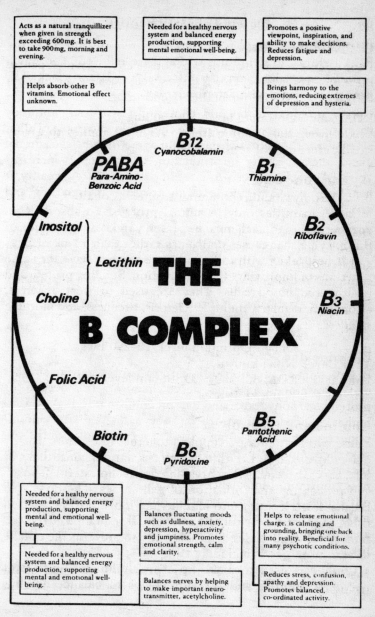

Figure 23

the Pill. For this reason, women often require 100 times the RDA before the symptoms of PMT are relieved. Too much protein, especially meat, also puts up B_6 needs, and a lack of B_6 is now associated with arteriosclerosis.

RDA: 2mg   Optimum level: 50–1000mg
Toxic level: 200–1000mg (the lower level applies to a very small percentage of sensitive people).

B_{12} and folic acid

B_{12} is the only vitamin containing a mineral, cobalt. B_{12} is found in large quantities only in animal protein. To absorb it an enzyme in the stomach must be present, and it is often a lack of this enzyme that causes deficiency rather than a lack of B_{12}.

It is best taken with folic acid since the two have the same functions of improving RNA production, building protein and healthy red blood cells. They are used to treat anaemia, alcoholism, diabetes, multiple sclerosis, tiredness, and morning sickness.

B_{12} – RDA: 2 mcg   Optimum level: 10–250 mcg
Toxic level: None known
Folic acid – RDA: 300 mcg   Optimum level: 400–4000 mcg
Toxic level: None known

Choline and inositol

These two nutrients are supplied together in lecithin, usually derived from soya. Lecithin, which is a natural constituent of bile, acts as an emulsifier, breaking down cholesterol deposits and preventing the formation of gall stones. The body also breaks down lecithin into choline and inositol to be used in other processes. Inositol acts as a natural tranquilliser and can replace valium in doses of 2g a day. It also prevents the uptake of various minerals including zinc.

Choline is used to make up acetylcholine, an important nerve transmitter, and therefore helps to balance nervous activity. Acetylcholine plays an important part in memory, and some studies have shown an increase in memory and intelligence when large amounts of choline and B_5 are supplemented.

Choline – RDA: Not established
Optimum level: 50–1000mg   Toxic level: None known
Inositol – RDA: Not established
Optimum level: 50–3000mg   Toxic level: None known

PABA and biotin

Biotin and PABA (Para Amino Benzoic Acid) have one thing in common: they are necessary for hair health. Biotin prevents hair loss, while PABA may prevent greying, PABA is also used as protection against sun burn, and may be needed to improve absorption of B_{12} and B_6.

PABA – RDA: Not established
Optimum level: 50–500mg   Toxic level: 2000mg daily
Biotin – RDA: Not established
Optimum level: 50–100mcg   Toxic level: None known

B_{13}, or orotic acid, a substance found in milk whey, has been reported to be effective in the treatment of multiple sclerosis. Another unrecognized vitamin is B_{17} or laetrile which is used to treat cancer. In Russia considerable attention has been focused on Pangamic acid or B_{15}, which is thought to facilitate oxygen transfer to the muscles. As time goes on, research results will determine whether or not these substances will join the list of essential nutrients.

Vitamin C ascorbic acid

Unlike all other vitamins, vitamin C is made by all animals except humans, apes and guinea pigs. For this reason leading authorities think that vitamin C isn't a vitamin after all. The theory is that we lost an enzyme needed to make ascorbic acid, perhaps at a time in our history when we ate a tropical diet containing much more vitamin C. As we were getting plenty in our diet, there was no need to use the energy consuming physiological process of transferring glucose to vitamin C. This gave us more mobility and put us at an advantage over other species. However, the climate is different now, and if current theories are correct we are all lacking in vitamin C. Colds, infections, allergies, arthritis and even an age span of only seventy years may all be the deficiency symptoms of too little vitamin C!

Whether we base our need for vitamin C on the amount that our ancestors would have obtained from eating a raw natural plant food diet, or the amount produced by an animal our size, the minimum requirement is 2300mg. In relation to other vitamins this is a lot, but vitamin C does a lot more than most. Firstly, it makes collagen, our intercellular glue, which supports bones, cartilage, skin and connective tissue. Secondly, it is essential for activating white blood cells, and also acts as an anti-bacterial and anti-viral agent. With proper use of vitamin C, colds and infections simply need not occur. Thirdly, like vitamin E, it is an anti-oxidant. It therefore protects other vitamins and fatty acids from destruction within the body. This is achieved by the ascorbic acid attaching to the harmful oxide and taking it out of the body. This it also does to carbon dioxide, mercury, DDT and even lead.

How much do you need?   Animals produce as much as three times the amount of vitamin C under conditions of stress, such as illness or overcrowding, and presumably we would too – if we could. Pollution, cigarettes, heat, the Pill, alcohol and many medical drugs also put up our need for this nutrient. To recommend 2g a day is conservative.

RDA: 30mg   Optimum level: 2–10g
Toxic level: None known

Vitamin P the bioflavanoids

Natural sources of vitamin C contain other substances known as the bioflavanoids or vitamin P. Together they are called vitamin C complex. The bioflavanoids have only one well known action: they are vital for the health and strength of our capillaries. As the capillaries are so small they can break without the right care. A tendency to bruise can therefore be a sign of deficiency. The bioflavanoids also act as ascorbic acid synergists. In other words they amplify and improve its efficiency.

RDA: Not established   Optimum level: 100–2000mg
Toxic level: None known

Nature always provides a solution,
To help us with our evolution.
It seems obvious to me,
We need vitamin C,
To combat excessive pollution.

DISCOVERING YOUR DEFICIENCIES

Choosing the right supplements for you is a personal affair. We each have different needs and these also change as you begin to correct your vitamin imbalances. However, there are three ways in which you can find out more exactly which vitamins are likely to help you.

The first way is by recognizing the body systems and organs that are most likely to need nutritional support. Are you a candidate for heart disease, or is digestion your sensitive area? The charts given earlier help you to choose the nutrients that may help you.

The second way is through blood tests, which are invasive, expensive, and not always conclusive. I only recommend these as a last resort.

The third and most useful way is to look at the signs and symptoms of deficiency that you may be experiencing. This next section lists a series of questions which help to pinpoint nutritional deficiency for the major vitamins.

Deficiency symptoms

Each question within this section starts with a list of symptoms associated with nutritional deficiency for a major vitamin. Underline the conditions that you often suffer from, and answer yes or no to the questions in each section.

VITAMIN A

Eye problems, bad eye sight, poor night vision, poor hearing, loss of smell, spots, dry flaky skin, oily skin, dandruff, mouth ulcers, throat infections, colds, diarrhoea, stuffy nose, stomach or duodenal ulcers, biliousness, depression, anger, frustration, warts, thrush, cystitis, sties, fatigue, loss of appetite.

Do you get more than three colds a year?

Are your eyes strained after long journeys?

VITAMIN D

Osteoarthritis, rheumatoid arthritis, rheumatism, rickets, middle backache, muscular numbness, tingling, spasm, lack of energy, tooth decay, hair loss, coarse hair, dry skin, near-sightedness, chillblains, weight problems.

Do you have pain and stiffness in the joints?

Do you have difficulty losing weight?

VITAMIN E

Hypertension, high blood pressure, chest pains, anaemia, loss of sex drive, rheumatic fever, diabetes, dry skin, easy bruising, infertility, slow wound healing, varicose veins, oedema, arteriosclerosis, weak heart, pancreatitis, puffy ankles

Do you get cramps after or during a long walk?

Do cuts take a long time to stop bleeding?

Do you get out of breath easily?

Is your pulse rate more than 75 per minute?

VITAMIN C

Colds, lack of energy, infections, allergies, arthritis, premature ageing, wrinkles, sagging skin, arteriosclerosis, shortness of breath, poor lactation, bad digestion, bleeding gums, cavities, bruising, painful and swollen joints, nose bleeds, slow wound healing, anaemia.

Do you live in a heavy traffic area?

Is your life style very stressful?

VITAMIN B COMPLEX

Confusion, irritability, depression, hair loss, premature grey hair, acne, bad skin, poor appetite, insomnia, neuritis, tension, difficulty relaxing, constipation, sleepiness after meals, allergies, hay fever, asthma.

Do you wake up tired?

Do you run out of energy easily?

Do you feel tense?

VITAMIN B$_1$

Tender muscles, stomach pains, constipation, slow irregular heart beat, prickly sensations in the legs, eye pains.

Do you have difficulty making decisions?

Are you losing weight?

Do you have difficulty breathing?

VITAMIN B$_2$

Bloodshot itchy eyes, burning or 'gritty' eyes, sore tongue, cracked lips, cataracts, eczema, dull oily hair, split nails, trembling, sluggishness, dizziness, inability to urinate, vaginal itching.

Are you sensitive to light?

VITAMIN B$_3$

Psychosis, schizophrenia, fatigue, acne, headaches, loss of appetite, migraines, bad breath, skin eruptions, insomnia, irritability, nausea, vomiting, tender gums, depression, rough inflamed skin, tremors, allergies, loss of memory, coated tongue.

Do you find it difficult to express your feelings?

Do you sometimes feel very energetic and overexcited?

Do you sometimes feel very depressed?

VITAMIN B$_5$

Apathy, abdominal pains, restlessness, vomiting, asthma, allergies, burning feet, muscle cramps, adrenal exhaustion, hypoglycaemia, exhaustion.

Do you find it hard to concentrate?

Do you sleep more than 10 hours a night?

VITAMIN B$_6$

Irritability, water retention, bloatedness, hypoglycaemia, depression, loss of hair, cracks around mouth and eyes, numbness, cramps in legs and arms, slow learning, morning sickness, postnatal depression, allergies, anaemia, nervousness, tingling hands, menopausal arthritis.

Do you have difficulty recalling your dreams?

Are you on the Pill?

If you answer 'yes' or underline more than 5 symptoms in each section, the chances are you could benefit from taking that vitamin. Make a list of the vitamins you could benefit from, and the appropriate dosage range from the vitamin chart. You'll need this for building your vitamin programme (see later). The most appropriate dosage to select initially is the lower value in the Optimum Range, although the dosage required will vary from person to person.

WHICH VITAMINS?

* The RDA, recommended daily amount, represents a level that protects against overt vitamin deficiency. The Optimum Level (OL) provides a range of supplementation, based on controlled research under medical supervision, that is safe and effective. These doses are not prescriptive.

Vitamin	What does it do?	How much?
A	Protects our 'inside skin', strengthening it against infection and ulcers, and outside skin, preventing spots. It helps slow down signs of ageing, helps prevent cancer, is good for the eyes, and is needed to make protein and sex hormones.	The need rises with a high protein diet or when recovering from infection. RDA: 2500 IU OL: 10,000 to 100,000 IU
D	Helps regulate the absorption and distribution of calcium, and is therefore essential for healthy bones and teeth.	RDA: 400 IUs OL: 400 to 4,000 IUs
E	Protects other substances in the body from oxidizing. This stops the destruction of unsaturated fats, hormones and vitamins, leaving the red blood cells supplied with pure oxygen, improving the functioning of the muscles. It also allows cells to function with less oxygen, and is beneficial for heart conditions and the skin.	People with high blood pressure or suspected heart conditions should not exceed 400 IUs. RDA: Not established OL: 400 to 4000 IUs.
F	Helps make adrenal, sex, and thyroid hormones and keeps the brain and nerves healthy. Found together with unsaturated fats,	RDA: Not established OL: 5 tablespoons

Vitamin	*What does it do?*	*How much?*
	these nutrients protect the skin, regulate blood coagulation, and dissolve cholesterol deposits.	
C	Makes collagen, our intercellular glue, improving condition of the skin and connective tissue. Also activates white blood cells, increasing our resistance to infection and viral invasion. Like vitamin E it protects other substances from oxidizing, and helps detoxify carbon dioxide, mercury, and lead.	Stress, pollution, cigarettes, the Pill, and alcohol increase the need for this vitamin. RDA: 30mg OL: 2 to 10g
B_1 Thiamine	It is needed to burn glucose in the cell, creating energy as well as making important nerve chemicals, toning the muscles of the digestive system, and helping in the breakdown of protein. Deficiency therefore affects digestion, energy, and the brain and nervous system.	Cooking and alcohol destroy B_1. RDA: 1.2mg OL: 25 to 250mg
B_2 Riboflavin	Helps neutralize acidity created when nutrients are burned for energy, reducing over-acidity symptoms like bloodshot, itchy eyes, dull oily hair, eczema, cataracts, and cracked lips. It is also essential for manufacturing the enzymes which break down fats, proteins, and carbohydrates.	B_2 is primarily destroyed by sunlight. RDA: 1.6mg OL: 25 to 250mg
B_3 Niacin	Involved in metabolism and the burning of sugars to form energy, the regulation of blood sugar and histamine levels, and helps keep down blood cholesterol. Because of its many roles it is useful in treating arteriosclerosis,	A 'blushing' sensation occurs with doses above 100mg. RDA: 18mg OL: 50 to 500mg

Vitamin	*What does it do?*	*How much?*
	arthritis, acne, depression, hypoglycaemia, alcoholism and headaches.	
B_5 Pantothenic Acid	Needed for energy production, fat and cholesterol synthesis, anti-body formation and manufacturing nerve chemicals. It also strengthens the adrenal glands and improves the production of cortisone, increasing resistance to stress.	RDA: Not established OL: 50 to 500mg
B_6 Pyridoxine	Makes hormones, enzymes, nerve chemicals and is needed for all metabolism. It also regulates sodium/potassium balance and can relieve symptoms of PMT. Also beneficial for morning sickness, postnatal depression, nervousness, hormone imbalances and allergies.	Cooking and the Pill destroy B_6. RDA: 2mg OL: 10 to 250mcg
B_{12} Cyanocobalamin	Needed for building protein and maintaining healthy red blood cells. It is used to treat anaemia, tiredness and morning sickness.	RDA: 2mcg OL: 10 to 250mcg
Lecithin	Contains choline, which balances the nerves, and inositol, a natural tranquillizer. Together they also act as an emulsifier, breaking down cholesterol deposits and preventing the formation of gall stones.	RDA: Not established OL: 1 to 5g

THE NUTRITIONAL MINERALS

Minerals are necessary for life and health. Some, such as calcium, magnesium, sodium, and potassium are required in large amounts, while others are needed in much smaller quantities, and are therefore called trace minerals. We obtain minerals from the food we eat, which in turn derives them from the soil or sea. Minerals in the soil are in an inorganic form and we cannot absorb them directly. However, plants can, incorporating them in their cell structure, which renders them absorbable by man. These are called organic minerals.

Largely due to the depletion of minerals in the soil, fresh foods no longer contain the sufficient amounts of some minerals, creating the need for mineral supplementation. To ensure correct absorption these minerals must be attached to an organic material such as an amino acid. These are called acid chelated minerals. Other good mineral chelators are orotate (B_{13}) and gluconate. Vitamin C helps iron absorption by keeping it in the reduced state. Some mineral supplements need to be chelated to ensure absorption. However, always check whether the quantity contained within the tablet is the total weight of the mineral and its chelator, or whether it is just the mineral. For example, 50mg of zinc orotate may only contain 5mg of zinc.

Calcium

The most abundant mineral in the body is calcium, and 99 per cent of this is in the bones and teeth. The remaining 1 per cent is needed for balanced nerve function, blood clotting, the heart muscles, and also for enzyme reactions. A lack of calcium can therefore result in osteoporosis, rickets, and contribute to the development of arthritic conditions. However, a hormone imbalance or lack of vitamin D can also disrupt the proper use of this mineral. Cramps, and irritability can be due to a lack of calcium, and this is probably the reason why hot milk drinks in the evening became popular, as the calcium they contain calms the nerves. While many foods contain small quantities of calcium, only milk products and sesame seeds contain sufficient amounts to easily meet daily requirements of 800mg or 1200mg for boys and girls between age 11 and 18, or pregnant and lactating women. A quarter pound of sesame seeds contain over 1000mg and a pint of milk (½ litre) contains some 600mg although some say that pasteurization renders the calcium less absorbable. The best form of calcium supplement is dolomite, because it also contains the right balance of magnesium, which works closely with calcium.

Optimum level: 700–1500mg

Magnesium

Named after the Greek city Magnesia, where large deposits of magnesium were found, this mineral is both needed and found in abundance in nature. We need it for the production of energy, muscle contraction, protein synthesis and the nervous system. It is also needed in a variety of enzyme reactions. Both toxicity and deficiency are rare, although the latter can occur with alcoholism, cirrhosis of the liver, and diabetes. Also, refining foods and cooking them dramatically reduces magnesium content. The daily requirement varies between 300mg and 500mg, which is found in milk, seeds, nuts, and wholegrains. Like calcium, dolomite is the best natural source of magnesium supplementation.

Optimum level: 300–500mg

Phosphorus

Phosphorus, like calcium, is essential for healthy bones and teeth. It is also found in every cell in your body, helping the breakdown of fats, carbohydrates and proteins, working with the muscles, and keeping blood and nerves healthy too. As phosphorus' functions are similar to that of calcium it is not surprising to find that a deficiency of one is generally accompanied by a deficiency of the other. For this reason sesame seeds are an excellent food as they contain both calcium and phosphorus. Pumpkin seeds, wheat germ, bran, and rice contain twice as much phosphorus as sesame seeds, and provided your diet contains plenty of calcium these, too, are excellent sources.

Optimum level: 100–500mg

Potassium

Potassium and sodium are both required in large amounts. Together they maintain the balance of water in the body, also being essential for nerves and muscles. Sodium is easily stored in the body, while much dietary potassium is excreted. For this reason it is important to get potassium on a daily basis. Also, excess sodium (salt) and diuretic drugs cause the loss of valuable potassium. Diets consisting of meat and little fruit or vegetables tend to lack potassium, while diets rich in green leafy vegetables, and fruit, with no added salt, are invariably well balanced. Bananas and dandelion coffee are especially high in potassium.

Optimum level: 10–100mg

Selenium

Since the discovery that cancer rates are low in areas with selenium rich soil, scientists have focused their attention on this fascinating trace element. Although the exact mechanism that helps selenium protect against cancer is not completely understood, it is thought that all antioxidants such as vitamin C and E have the same beneficial effect.

Selenium and vitamin E are also involved in maintaining healthy capillaries. While vitamin E prevents the formation of toxic by-products of fats, which can destroy the walls of capillaries, selenium acts as a second line of defence destroying these toxins in the blood. Provided there is sufficient vitamin E, this second line of defence is not needed simply because there are no toxic fat by-products in the blood, but any lack of vitamin E makes selenium a very important element for maintaining healthy capillaries.

Optimum level: 20–100mcg

Zinc

The importance of zinc for good nutrition is becoming increasingly realized. Like many other minerals, the levels of zinc in the 'average' diet are small, because of food refining and processing, pollution and antagonistic drugs. Cadmium, a pollutant from car exhaust, and the Pill rapidly deplete zinc from the body. Stress also has the same effect.

Zinc is needed for proper bone growth and is of particular importance in the development of sex organs. Since the highest concentration is in the prostate gland it has been theorized that males cease to grow as fast as females in their early teens because the dietary zinc is used to develop sex glands, leaving an insufficient amount for other growth processes. It also speeds up wound healing, mobilizes vitamin A from the liver, and is good for treating arteriosclerosis. Zinc also slows down the action of insulin given to diabetics, decreasing their need for this drug, thereby helping to maintain normal blood sugar balance.

The most common signs of deficiency are white spots or lines under the nails, brittle nails, inability to taste foods, and a lack of appetite. If these symptoms are present it is wise to take a zinc supplement, together with vitamin B_6 which improves utilization. People with psoriasis require much more than 15 mg of zinc, and since zinc levels are lowest a week before menstruation, premenstrual syndrome often stops with zinc and B_6 supplementation. Foods which are high in zinc are fish and shellfish, especially herring and oysters, while grains, peas, eggs, and yeast contain a lesser amount.

Optimum level: 10–50mg

Manganese

Like zinc, manganese helps normalize blood sugar levels and is therefore important for diabetics. It is involved with other stages of sugar metabolism as well as fat metabolism, and is needed to make a variety of enzymes. Manganese also balances nervous activity and hormone production both in the pituitary gland, and thyroid where it is needed to produce the hormone thyroxin. Deficiency symptoms are not clear in humans, although in animals, defects relating to bone growth are apparent. Since it is removed in refining flours and is commonly deficient in soil it is important to eat wholegrains, especially bran, green leafy and root vegetables, and fruit.

Optimum level: 2.5–5.0mg

Iron

Most people associate iron with anaemia. For this reason more people take iron supplements than any other mineral. Yet anaemia results from deficiency of B_6, B_{12}, folic acid or zinc as well as iron. As a result of this popular misconception many people take too much iron which is toxic in large amounts.

Iron combines with protein to make haemoglobin, a major constituent of blood cells. While iron is recycled within the body, excessive bleeding, mostly caused by menstruation, can deplete iron levels causing iron deficiency anaemia. In these cases iron supplements are beneficial. Dietary sources are meat, especially organ meats, deep green leafy vegetables, wholegrains, fruits, fish and molasses.

Optimum level: 10–50mg

Chromium

The discovery that chromium is released into the bloodstream when the blood sugar level goes up, confirms its important role in helping insulin to control blood sugar levels. It is combined in the liver with B_3 and two amino acids to make Glucose Tolerance Factor (GTF).

Since any conditions which cause an increase in blood sugar, for example eating sugar and cakes, or coffee, also use up chromium, this mineral is often deficient in those eating refined food diets. Chromium supplementation is also effective in treating hypoglycaemics and diabetics. The dietary sources are brewer's yeast, whole grains, beef, mushrooms, and molasses.

Optimum level: 20–200mcg

DETOXIFYING THE TOXIC MINERALS

The idea that society would choose to poison itself merely for industrial ease and financial gain, seems strange. Yet this is the situation regarding lead, a powerful neurotoxin. Largely due to the presence of lead in petrol, British children living in cities commonly take in, through their food and the air they breathe, higher levels of lead than the World Health Organization deems safe. The effects of such excesses of lead are hyperactivity, aggression, disturbed behaviour, lessened intelligence, and difficulty sleeping, resulting in fatigue. In short, lead is as great a social phenomenon as alcohol, the only difference being that lead intoxication is not voluntary.

´Only the politics behind lead, through its use in raising the octane level in petrol, and our conservatism, has allowed the current dangerous levels in our environment to continue. While official bodies in Britain do recognize the problem, they understate the number of people affected by lead intoxication. Since the first signs of most neurotoxins reveal themselves as impaired mentation and emotional instability, it is hard to measure the size of the problem we are dealing with.

In my London Clinic approximately 20 per cent of patients have excess lead levels, determined through hair mineral analysis. Of these, a number are young children who often show signs of hyperactivity, disturbed sleep, fussiness about eating, and aggressive outbursts.

The Needleman study in Birmingham compared teachers' ratings of pupils for distractibility, non-persistence, dependence, disorganization, hyperactivity, frustration, daydreaming, as well as ability on a number of tasks. They then divided the children into six groups, from high dentine lead levels to low. On each rating the higher the lead level in the group, the worse the rating. There was even a significant difference in IQ of some 5 points between those with high and low lead.

Detoxifying lead

Of course the real answer is to remove lead from petrol, which I hope will happen in the next two years. But meanwhile there are some easy and safe ways to protect yourself from excess toxic metals, including lead.

Because lead is taken into the bones, where it can later be released and taken to the brain via the bloodstream, it is important to keep your calcium levels high. This helps to prevent the initial uptake of lead. Vitamin C, zinc, and alginic acid from seaweed, as well as pectin from apples, all help to carry lead out of the body. This has been shown to be effective in a number of studies, some of which used battery manufacturers, who are frequently exposed to very dangerous levels of lead. Another study by Pfeiffer treated psychiatric patients with high lead levels using only vitamin C and zinc and found a significant decrease in lead levels, dropping 25 per cent over a two month period.

For this reason I asked supplement manufacturers to make a supplement that contained the right balance of vitamin C, zinc, and alginic acid. This supplement is now available and is called Detox. If you can't get it in your local health food shop, ring or write to Health + Plus Ltd, 118 Station Road, Chinnor, Oxon OX9 4WZ (Tel: 0844 52098). The recommended dose is 1 for children under 10, 2 for adolescents under 15, and up to 5 for adults. It is also a good idea to eat plenty of apples, as these also help to remove excess lead.

Cadmium and mercury

Another highly toxic metal is cadmium. Like lead it is found in car exhaust fumes, as well as paint, cigarettes, tin cans, tea and coffee, and some industrial processes. Fortunately, cadmium toxicity is rare — however, since it can store in the body over a long period in time, slight but long term exposure can lead to toxicity 50 years later. One of the conditions associated with cadmium toxicity is emphysema. The Detox formula can again help protect against this metal since zinc is an antagonist of cadmium and prevents its uptake.

Mercury poisoning is very rare and is usually due to occupational exposure. As the clinical symptoms (which include tingling, headaches, fatigue, visual, hearing and speech defects, paralysis and convulsions) are irreversible, it is important to pick up early signs which are forgetfulness, fatigue, and headaches.

Unless there is a possibility of industrial exposure a high mercury level is most likely due to consumption of food stuffs contaminated with mercury. High sources other than industrial are coal burning, pesticides, fungicides, large fish (e.g. tuna), batteries, paints, and cosmetics.

The sulphur containing amino acids, which are found in onions and garlic, help protect against mercury. The Detox formula together with a selenium supplement provide an even safer insurance against this metal.

Aluminium

Excessive levels of aluminium are quite common due to our usage of this metal for making many household products. Extremely high amounts are likely to cause symptoms such as gastrointestinal irritation, rickets, and psoriasis, as well as being linked to cystic fibrosis and senility.

Such exposure can occur due to frequent use of aluminium cookware, aluminium foil, aluminium salt (most table salts), toothpaste, cigarette filters, processed cheese, cosmetics and pharmaceuticals. Many antacid tablets contain aluminium salts, which should be marked on the label, and are therefore best avoided. Apart from taking Detox, it is wise to supplement with B_6, and keep down your intake of high phosphorus-containing foods, if you have high levels of aluminium. The next section explains how you can find your levels of both toxic and nutritional minerals using Hair Mineral Analysis.

WHICH MINERALS? – A GUIDE TO HAIR MINERAL ANALYSIS

Although less is generally known about minerals, they are no less important than vitamins for maintaining our health. In fact, since so little is publicized about these essential micro-nutrients, many farming procedures and food processing methods are allowed to rob us of these valuable nutrients. Fortunately for us, a new scientific procedure for analyzing mineral levels, without the invasion of blood tests or the unreliability and awkwardness of urine tests, is now available and that is hair mineral analysis.

Hair mineral analysis can be carried out using one of three techniques. These are atomic absorption, atomic emission, and X-ray fluorescence. Each technique has its advantages and disadvantages, however, suffice it to say that accurate results can be produced by a trained technician, using a combination of two of these methods. The reason for this, for example, is that X-ray fluorescence is good for measuring most minerals except calcium, magnesium, sodium and potassium, so a good laboratory would use atomic absorption for these minerals.

In the case of X-ray fluorescence, the hair sample, which must always be taken from the first inch and a half of hair close to the scalp, is then washed many times to remove particles that have settled on the hair. It is then dissolved in acid, and when in a solution form, is placed in a grid which goes into a machine called an X-ray spectroscope. Here it is bombarded with X-rays which bounce off the sample at different angles depending on the amount of each mineral in the hair. Another machine counts the amount of radiation coming off at each angle and therefore works out the amount of 14 toxic and nutritional minerals in the hair.

How reliable is hair mineral analysis?

Many people have assumed that the levels of minerals in the hair directly reflect the levels in the body. Unfortunately, like most chemical tests, interpretation isn't that straightforward. Others have claimed that you can diagnose serious illness in advance from hair mineral analysis. I am sure that in the not too distant future it will be possible to use this inexpensive technique to pinpoint specific illnesses. However at the moment, we can only rely on hair mineral analysis to pinpoint mineral excess or deficiencies. One of the great advantages of this technique is that it gives a reflection of how our body has been functioning over three months, since that is the time it takes to produce up to the first two inches of hair. It is this long term information that has made many nutritionists and doctors turn away from the laborious procedure of blood tests.

However, when a mineral is being incorrectly used in the body it can be excreted into the hair giving a false high reading of that mineral, when the cells are still deficient. For this reason it is most important to interpret the results of hair mineral analyses very carefully.

How to interpret hair mineral analysis

The hair mineral chart below contains suggested *optimum* nutrient ranges designed to promote optimum health. The first two minerals are calcium and magnesium. Since these two minerals tend to wash into the hair, elevated levels need not indicate excess. Low levels of either are a cause of concern and should be rectified. A high ratio of calcium to magnesium often indicates a lack of magnesium which can negatively affect the uptake of calcium. So this too would warrant correction. A low ratio is correlated to glucose intolerance, especially if low chromium and low manganese is also present. A ratio of 15:1

has been frequently found with people with multiple food allergies.

Regarding the balance between sodium and potassium, these minerals tend to wash out of the hair and therefore low levels of both are not uncommon. This need not indicate imbalance unless there are associated signs of deficiency. Extremely high levels of both usually indicates a metabolic disturbance such as disturbed protein synthesis or kidney problems. High sodium low potassium is an indication to reduce dietary sodium.

Low iron levels in the hair will not always mean low levels in the blood and therefore this test is not accurate for diagnosing anaemia. However, a level below 0.5 or above 4 is suspicious. In such an event it would be wise to have a blood test and examine your diet.

A high level of copper, especially if accompanied by a low zinc level, can be brought down with zinc, and vitamin C. A low copper level reflects low copper, as has been shown in studies which have monitored copper level dropping through pregnancy.

A high zinc level does not always mean excess zinc. A study involving hyperactive children found very high hair levels, while diets were very deficient. This indicates a disturbance of zinc utilization, causing zinc to be deposited in the hair. Since high hair levels do not usually indicate high body levels it is alright to supplement with zinc provided the level is below 33mg%, and provided copper isn't low, since zinc is a copper antagonist. Pfeiffer thinks a lack of B_6 can prevent uptake of zinc and can be responsible for false high readings. Taking B_6 often balances zinc levels.

Manganese is very deficient in British diets and therefore requires supplementation if hair levels are too low.

A low cobalt level gives some indication of B_{12} deficiency since this vitamin contains cobalt.

Low chromium together with a high calcium:magnesium ratio and low manganese is a fairly reliable sign of impaired glucose tolerance.

Figure 24

BIOLAB MEDICAL UNIT.

THE STONE HOUSE,
9 WEYMOUTH STREET,
LONDON, W1N 3FF.

TELEPHONE 01 636 5959
01 636 5905

HAIR MINERAL ANALYSIS REPORT.

PATIENT:

REFERENCE NUMBER: 309488

AGE: 40
DATE: 21-03-1988

DOCTOR:

SEX: MALE
SAMPLE DATE: 15-03-1988

HEIGHT:
HAIR COLOUR: DARK BROWN
CONDITIONER:
HIGHLIGHT:
TINT:

WEIGHT:
SHAMPOO: VARIES
BLEACH:
PERM:

(ALL RESULTS IN PARTS PER MILLION)

	REFERENCE RANGE:	RESULTS:	LOW	REFERENCE RANGE	HIGH	
CALCIUM	200 - 600	525				Ca
MAGNESIUM	30 - 95	22				Mg
PHOSPHORUS*	100 - 210	167				P
SODIUM*	90 - 340	77				Na
POTASSIUM*	50 - 120	32				K
IRON*	20 - 60	34				Fe
COPPER	10 - 40	19				Cu

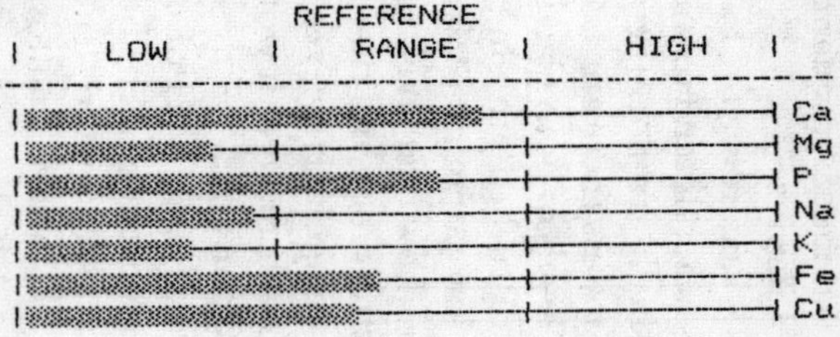

ZINC	150	-	240	144
CHROMIUM	0.6	-	1.5	0.68
MANGANESE	1.0	-	2.6	0.9
SELENIUM	1.5	-	4.0	1.8
NICKEL	0.4	-	1.4	0.72
COBALT*	0.1	-	0.7	0.40

Zn Cr Mn Se Ni Co

* Clinical significance of hair concentration of asterisked elements has not been established.

	ACCEPT	RAISED	TOXIC			
				TOXIC RESULT	ACCEPTABLE | RAISED | TOXIC	
LEAD	<15	15 - 40	>40	4.5		Pb
MERCURY	<2.0	2.0 - 5.0	>5.0	0.31		Hg
CADMIUM	<0.5	0.5 - 2.0	>2.0	0.14		Cd
ARSENIC	<2.0	2.0 - 5.0	>5.0	0.12		As
ALUMINIUM	<10.0	10.0- 25.0	>25.0	2.7		Al

RATIO:	MIDLINE:	RESULT:
Ca/Mg	6.1:1	23.8
Ca/P	2.6:1	3.1
Na/K	2.3:1	2.4
Zn/Cu	8.5:1	7.5

RATIO:	NORMAL:	RESULT:
Zn/Pb	>40:1	32
Zn/Cd	>400:1	1028
Se/Cd	>3.4:1	12.8
Se/Hg		5.8

Magnesium, zinc and (mild) manganese deficiencies.

Analysis by John Howard D.Sc.   Dr Stephen Davies, Medical Director.

The toxic minerals are quite straightforward. A high level in the hair indicates toxic exposure. It is wise to begin detoxification using the appropriate procedure described in the section called Detoxifying Toxic Minerals.

The only times when false high readings can occur is with certain hair care treatments which are known to contain minerals which stay on the hair, and some dandruff shampoos which contain arsenic. Arsenic is very inabsorbable so high hair levels, which are in themselves rare, are usually due to outside contamination and not some plot to poison you!

An analysis of your hair can be obtained through the Institute for Optimum Nutrition for £25. They can be contacted by writing to ION, 5 Jerdan Place, London SW6 1BE, or telephoning 01 385 7984. They analyse 22 minerals, including calcium, magnesium, sodium, potassium, iron, copper, zinc, chromium, manganese, selenium, cobalt, nickel, vanadium, lead, arsenic, cadmium, mercury, and aluminium. They also provide a personal five page interpretation with each hair analysis.

Symptoms of deficiency or excess

Unfortunately, minerals are not as easy as vitamins to pinpoint from their deficiency symptoms, since so many of the symptoms can be a result of other nutritional deficiences too. However, here is a chart which lists the symptoms associated with each mineral, how the mineral works, and which foods contain high levels of each mineral.

NUTRITIONAL MINERALS

Mineral	Rich food sources	Action
Calcium	Milk, cheese, sesame seeds, oats, millet, kelp, nuts, fresh vegetables.	The most abundant mineral in the body; 99 per cent is in bones and teeth. One per cent needed for balanced

Mineral	Rich food sources	Action
		nerve function, healthy blood clotting, heart muscles, enzyme reactions. Deficiency can lead to tooth decay, fragile bones, muscle and menstrual cramps, brittle nails, nervousness, headaches, eczema and rheumatoid arthritis.
Magnesium	Nuts, soya beans, whole grains, green leafy vegetables (not spinach), sesame seeds.	Needed for producing energy, muscle contraction, regulating nervous system, protein synthesis. Lack can produce depression, poor memory, irritability, nervous disorders, muscle tremors.
Sodium	Sea salt, celery, olives, meats, vegetables. (An abundance of salt is often found in prepared and processed food.)	Excess leads to fluid retention, loss of potassium, high blood pressure, stomach ulcers, bronchial asthma.
Potassium	Vegetables, fruits, wheatgerm, bananas, avocados, dandelion coffee, prunes, whole grains, nuts.	Symptoms of deficiency include muscle weakness, tiredness, constipation, poor reflexes, nervous disorders, arthritis.
Iron	Liver, lean beef, egg yolk, beans, lentils, dried fruit, yeast, whole grains.	Helps transport oxygen to cells. Deficiency associated with anaemia, weakness, pale skin, constipation, kidney damage, flatulence, thin nails and excessive levels of lead.
Copper	Shellfish (especially oysters), organ meats, whole cereals, dried fruit, almonds, green vegetables.	Copper in small amounts is essential for health. High levels of copper, however, are considered toxic. Deficiency is uncommon

Mineral	Rich food sources	Action
		because of abundance in present environment. Low levels associated with weakness, anaemia, arthritis, skin sores, hair loss, digestive disorders. High levels: hardening of arteries, kidney disease, psychosis, early senility.
Zinc	Wheatgerm, pumpkin and sunflower seeds, yeast, eggs, oysters, nuts, sprouted grains, wholewheat bread.	Required for satisfactory bone growth, sexual development, energy production, maintenance of blood sugar levels. Also needed to use Vitamins A and B_6 effectively. Deficiency symptoms may show in stretch marks, irregular menstrual cycle, impotence, prolonged wound healing, joint pain, loss of appetite, white fingernail spots, and dandruff.
Chromium	Brewer's yeast, whole grains, liver, beef, mushrooms, molasses (lost in refined sugar).	Deficiencies associated with arteriosclerosis, improper glucose metabolism, hypoglycaemia, diabetes, heart disease, improper fat metabolism.
Manganese	Green leafy vegetables, pineapple, bran, wheat, kelp, egg yolk, nuts, seeds.	Helps normalize blood sugar levels. Involved in stages of sugar and fat metabolism; needed to produce enzymes, hormones, pituitary and thyroid gland; balances nervous activity. Deficiency associated with lack of sex drive, dizziness, convulsions, rheumatoid arthritis, nervous instability in pregnancy.

Mineral	Rich food sources	Action
Selenium	Brewer's yeast, tuna, herring, wheatgerm, bran, whole grains, broccoli, onion, garlic, tomatoes.	Protects arteries by destroying toxins in blood which can damage artery walls. Currently under scrutiny – lack of selenium may cause cancer; its presence may be linked with healthy old age.
Nickel	Buckwheat, oats, rye, cabbage, spinach, green leafy vegetables.	Possibly associated with cirrhosis of the liver and chronic kidney failure. Deficiencies likely in diets high in fat, refined carbohydrates and dairy produce.
Cobalt	Lean beef, organ meats, tuna, haddock, milk, cottage cheese, eggs, chicken.	Vitamin B_{12} contains cobalt and a lack of B_{12} results in anaemia. Deficiency symptoms related to cobalt alone are not yet established.
Vanadium	Whole cereals, nuts, root vegetables.	Deficiency symptoms not yet clearly established, but its value to man comes from the knowledge that animals get high cholesterol levels when vanadium is low in their diet.

TOXIC MINERALS

Mineral	Rich food sources	Action
Lead	Non-food sources include car exhaust, cigarettes, lead-based paint.	Toxic symptoms include depression, irritability, apathy, confusion, hyperactivity, behaviour problems in children, digestive disorders, nausea, loss of appetite, muscle weakness, insomnia.

Mineral	Rich food sources	Action
Mercury	Large fish (e.g. tuna). Non-food sources include pesticides, fungicides, some paints.	Mercury poisoning usually due to occupational exposure. Symptoms include tingling sensations, headaches, fatigue, visual, hearing and speech defects, forgetfulness.
Cadmium	Refined and canned foods. Non-food sources include cigarettes, detergents, fertilizers.	Toxic symptoms include hypertension, hardening of the arteries, strokes, kidney or liver damage. Cadmium can be stored in the body over years of exposure.
Arsenic	Some table salts, some beers and wines. Non-food sources include pesticides, some dyes and paints.	High arsenic levels uncommon since it is easily excreted from the body. High level symptoms, however, include nausea, poor wound healing, sore throats, loss of hair and nails.
Aluminium	Some table salts and processed cheeses. Non-food sources include aluminium cookware and foil, toothpaste, cigarette filters.	Possible signs of high amounts: gastrointestinal irritation, rickets, psoriasis.

NUTRIENTS FOR A HEALTHY PREGNANCY

Pregnancy is a time when nutrition is doubly important. Despite this fact many women are cautious about supplementing vitamins and minerals during pregnancy. However, certain vitamins and minerals are needed in relatively large amounts to maximise the chances of a healthy pregnancy and a healthy child. A deficiency in the B vitamin folic acid has been linked with an increased risk for spina bifida. However, the mother need not even be showing deficiency signs of folic acid to be supplying too low levels to her child. Needs for B_6, B_{12}, biotin and the minerals zinc, iron, calcium and magnesium also increase during pregnancy. The following amounts supplemented on top of a good diet are recommended during pregnancy: B_6 100mg, B_{12} 25mcg, folic acid 200mcg, biotin 100mcg, calcium 200mg, magnesium 100mg, zinc 17.5mg, iron 12mg.

However, the best time to start supplementing is before pregnancy. The most critical time for nutrition is one month before pregnancy (when the female ovum is maturing) and the first three months of pregnancy. It is also important not to smoke or drink alcohol during this time and throughout the whole of pregnancy.

NUTRITION FOR HEALTHY CHILDREN

Good nutrition is especially important during the first fourteen years of life. It is during this time that the body is growing and maturing, and the correct supply of nutrients makes all the difference. During these formative years nutrition can affect physical growth and size, intelligence, and resistance to disease – for life. From adolescence onwards, for example, the strength of your immune system starts to decline. The speed at which this happens depends on how good your nutrition was in childhood. The most important nutrients are those involved in growth, those involved in skeletal development and those involved in brain function.

Going for growth
We grow by making and maturing new cells. These cells are

25 per cent protein. So an adequate supply of protein is essential. But more essential are the catalysts needed to turn protein from food into highly complex cells. These are vitamin A, vitamin B_6, B_{12}, folic acid and zinc. Children need relatively more of these nutrients, but sadly most children do not get enough. In one study in which the diets of 90 schoolchildren in a comprehensive school were analysed the majority of children didn't even get the basic Recommended Daily Allowance of vitamin B_6, folic acid and zinc.

Since zinc is involved in the utilization of vitamin A, many children also do not get adequate vitamin A nutrition. The RDA is 2250 IU. However, a healthy diet similar to that which our ancestors would have eaten would provide ten times this amount mainly from the vegetarian form of vitamin A, beta-carotene. This is richly provided in carrots, oranges, beetroot and apricots.

WHAT'S MISSING IN OUR CHILDREN'S DIETS?

Nutrient	Percentage of RDA supplied in average child's diet	
	25% 50% 75% 100%	
Vitamin B_6		88%
Folic Acid		61%
Vitamin E		100%
Calcium		56%
Magnesium		68%
Zinc		44%
Iron		37%
Manganese		47%

Vitamin B_6 is found in foods that contain protein. This is a clever natural design since B_6 is needed both in the digestion and use of protein. The problem is that we, unlike our ancestors, cook most protein-rich foods and thereby destroy some of the vitamin B_6. Foods rich in B_6 are wholegrains, beans, especially butter beans, fish, meat, avocado, banana and wheatgerm.

Vitamin B_{12} is only found in animal produce, including eggs and milk products. Folic acid is in all green leafy vegetables. Again, it is easily destroyed by cooking, so eating something raw is essential.

Zinc is needed for the formation of the RNA molecule. This clever molecule is like the foreman on a building site. It reads the plan for making cells, called DNA, and assembles the necessary ingredients, including proteins, to make new cells. Any food that is actively growing, or any seed which contains the potential for growth will contain zinc. It is, therefore, richest in meat, fish and other animal produce, and is also abundant in wheatgerm, whole grains, sprouts and seeds. It is perhaps the most commonly deficient mineral for children. This may be due to overfarming depleting our soil of zinc – as well as to poor dietary habits.

Making strong bones and teeth

Bones and teeth are made out of a matrix of protein into which goes calcium, magnesium and phosphorus. Children need plenty of these minerals to develop strong bones and healthy teeth. However, the process of using calcium, which is the most important of these three minerals, depends on many factors other than dietary intake. For example, vitamin D turns into a hormone that helps lay down calcium. Deficiency in vitamin D, too much protein, a lack of exercise, a high sugar or fat diet are all factors that hinder calcium absorption. Vitamin D, calcium and magnesium are commonly deficient. While milk is a good source of calcium it is a very poor source of magnesium. Only green leafy vegetables, nuts and seeds contain significant quantities of both these minerals. The best vegetables are the crunchy ones with a strong structure, like cauliflower, kale and cabbage. The best seeds are sesame and sunflower seeds, and the best nuts are almonds and brazils. Vitamin D is in eggs, milk and meat. In children on a semi-vegetarian diet it is worth supplementing vitamin D as well as calcium and magnesium. Phosphorus is well supplied in most diets.

How to boost your child's intelligence

Your child's intelligence depends in part upon good nutrition, and protection from anti-nutrients like lead. To illustrate this, one study in America found that intelligence at age three correlated to lead levels at birth. The higher the lead level the lower the intelligence. It is now well known that head circumference of babies, which is related to brain development, is greater in babies with high levels of zinc and low levels of cadmium and lead. Another trial involving 12- and 13-year-olds found that giving a daily vitamin and mineral supplement increased non-verbal IQ scores by, on average, 10 per cent!

The brain is an unbelievable organ containing millions of special nerve cells. Each nerve cell can connect with 10,000 others and ends up looking like a tree shooting out roots and branches. It is known that high lead levels can decrease the number of connections. It is very likely that the intake of important nutrients determines the level of intelligence. The key nutrients are all those involved in growth, vitamin A, B_6, B_{12}, folic acid and zinc, and also calcium, magnesium, choline, pantothenic acid (vitamin B_5), and essential fatty acids.

Nerve cells communicate by sending electrical messages. These electrical messages occur because of fluctuations in electrically charged minerals, predominantly sodium, potassium, chlorine, calcium and magnesium. It is only calcium and magnesium that are commonly deficient. The ability to turn on or off electrical stimulation depends upon neurotransmitters. There are many different kinds of neurotransmitters most of which are protein-like substances. For example, one neurotransmitter, serotonin, rises in the evening and brings on sleep. It is made from the amino acid tryptophan, in the presence of adequate vitamin B_3 and B_6. Another, adrenalin, rises as light enters through the translucent portions of our skull, waking us up. Adrenalin is made from tyrosine, an amino acid found in food.

The most important neurotransmitter of all is acetylcholine.

This requires choline and vitamin B_5 for its production. Although choline can be made by the body we receive significant amounts from our diets. We may not be able to make enough to maximize brain function and so rely on a dietary intake. It is classified as a semi-essential nutrient. In both human and animal studies, giving large amounts of choline or vitamin B_5 causes measurable improvement in intelligence and memory. In one study in Britain twelve intelligent, working women were given 500mg of choline and 500mg of vitamin B_5 every day for three months. At the end of three months their intelligence had risen by 15 per cent! Choline, which is rich in fish, and vitamin B_5 are also important for children of all ages.

Most people think of fat as bad for them, but children need an adequate supply of the right kind of fat. Hundreds of cases of children failing to thrive have been put down to over-health-conscious parents keeping their children on a low fat diet. The kind of fat that children need is unsaturated fat provided in nuts, seeds and vegetable oils. Fat is used to make myelin, the insulating layer around nerves. With all these new brain cells there's a tremendous need for plenty of good insulation. In fact one third of the brain is fat. It is also needed to make prostaglandins, hormone-like substances found in large amounts in the brain. So it is important not to go overboard with low-fat diets for children. In practical terms this means whole milk instead of skimmed, eating nuts and seeds, and the use of unsaturated fats including olive oil, cheese and eggs. However, it is still best to stay off fried foods, lots of fatty meat and junk foods high in fat.

Keeping children sugar free

The taste for sugar is an acquired habit. We all like the taste of sweetness, but research has shown that only those who eat a high sugar diet like high levels of sugar in their diet. So it is vitally important to keep children on a less sweet diet. This good habit may be with them for life. The best way to do this is to gradually lower the sweetness of everything they eat including 'health' foods. For example, if you give your child pure fruit juice start diluting this until your child gets used to half water, half juice, or two thirds water one third juice. Also cut down the intake of dried fruit choosing fresh fruit instead.

Of course, there are always special occasions when it's just about impossible to be sugar free, for instance at birthday parties. The secret is to make delicious sugar-free cakes and dishes as an alternative. You may choose to use a little honey or dried fruit, but as long as the end-product is less sweet than the multi-coloured alternative, you're making a difference.

The trouble with sugar is that no one can really say that the odd spoonful actually harms your health. Sugar is completely devoid of all vitamins and minerals needed to digest and metabolize it, so it does effectively lower body stores of these vital nutrients. But the problem with sugar is that the taste for it is habit forming. Before long your child may be getting 20 per cent of his or her calories from sugar, most of which is hidden in snacks. So start by getting sugar-free cereal, using fruit as a sweetener, and if necessary give low sugar sweets as well as nuts and fruit for snacks at school. There are many sugar-free sweets available nowadays in health food shops.

Additives – who needs them?

Many children consume as much as 10lb of food additives and preservatives each year. The vast majority of these chemicals have been used in foods for less than 15 years. We simply have no idea what their long-term consequences are on health. What we do know is that children are far more susceptible to the damaging effects of additives. For this reason some additives are not advised for children's foods. Many manufacturers get round this restriction by not stating that their product is for children. But one has to question who else would eat a multi-coloured trifle decorated with silver balls!

The most harmful additives are the food colourings such as tartrazine, which is used to colour drinks and foods orange. The colours have E numbers from E100 to E180. With so many additive-free foods available nowadays it is quite possible to keep children additive free.

Brain pollution

Children up to age twelve have higher levels of lead and some other toxic metals than adults. In childhood, levels peak between the ages of three and six. This is probably due to their handling things and putting objects in their mouths, as well as being lower to the ground where lead levels are higher. Because children's brains are still developing they are particularly effected by toxic metals. The average lead level known to affect intelligence and behaviour in children is 12mcg/dl. The average lead level of a child in Britain is 16mcg/dl.

It's impossible to avoid all these pollutants but it is possible to limit exposure and minimize absorption (see the chapter on Detoxifying Toxic Minerals). The minerals calcium and zinc, and vitamin C all prevent the uptake of lead and promote its excretion from the body. It is vital to ensure an adequate supply of these nutrients.

Keeping your child immune

Young children are especially prone to infections. To an extent this is unavoidable since it takes years to develop a strong immune system. It is also necessary to become infected with some diseases in order to develop immunity. However, the severity, length and frequency of such infections depends on nutritional status. There are many nutrients that are essential for the immune system. These include vitamins A, C, E, B, calcium, magnesium, zinc and selenium. Of these, vitamin A and zinc are perhaps the most important. It is precisely these two nutrients that are also needed for growth, and it is these that are so often deficient in the diets of children. During times of infections it is wise to supplement two or three times the optimal level (shown later) until the infection is over.

Supplements for children

According to Dr Roger Williams, often called the founder of optimum nutrition, 'The greatest hope for increasing [health and] lifespan can be offered if nutrition – from the time of pre-natal development up to old age – is continuously of the highest quality.' Although diet is crucial and the right place to start, every child can benefit from proper vitamin and mineral supplementation.

The ideal daily intake of these nutrients, assuming an already good diet, is shown opposite. The chart shows ideal intakes of each nutrient from 0 to 14. After age 14 nutrient intakes are little different from those recommended for adults. These are not based on RDAs but on optimal levels.

One of the major difficulties in getting the right supplements for your child is availability. Most children's vitamins are chewable and designed to taste nice, for obvious reasons. The trouble is that zinc tastes bitter and calcium tastes chalky. So most children's chewables do not contain anywhere near enough of these two nutrients. The only chewable supplement that I know to contain good amounts of these, and other nutrients is a product called Supermouse, made by Health+Plus Ltd. Unlike many chewables it is sweetened with a very small amount of fructose and contains only natural flavourings. The recommended dose for a six-year-old provides 9mg of zinc, and 225mg of calcium, compared to our recommendations of 10mg of zinc and 900mg of calcium. So there's a considerable shortfall in calcium. This can be made up by giving your child a calcium-rich diet. For example, a breakfast of yoghurt, two dessertspoons of ground sesame seeds, wheatgerm and banana already provides 400mg of calcium. You can also supplement your child's diet by adding calcium powder, available from most chemists, to some food, or by giving them a dolomite

OPTIMUM DAILY INTAKES FROM AGE ONE TO FOURTEEN

Nutrient Vitamins	Less than 1	Age 1	2	3–4	5–6	7–8	9–11	12–14
A	4,000 IU	4,500	5,000	5,500	6,000	7,000	7,500	10,000
D	400 IU	400	400	400	400	400	400	400
E	20 IU	20	25	30	35	45	60	80
C	100 mg	100	200	300	400	500	600	700
B₁ (thiamine)	5 mg	5	6	8	12	16	20	25
B₂ (riboflavin)	5 mg	5	6	8	12	16	20	25
B₃ (niacin)	7 mg	10	14	16	18	20	22	25
B₅ (pantothenic acid)	10 mg	10	15	20	25	30	35	40
B₆ (pyridoxine)	5 mg	5	7	10	12	16	20	25
B₁₂	5 mcg	6	7	8	9	10	10	10
Folic Acid	100 mcg	100	120	140	160	180	200	250
Biotin	150 mcg	150	180	210	240	270	300	300
Minerals								
Sodium	3,000 mg	3,000	3,000	3,000	3,000	3,000	3,000	3,000
Potassium	3,000 mg	3,500	3,750	4,000	4,250	4,500	5,000	5,000
Calcium	600 mg	600	700	800	900	1,000	1,100	1,100
Magnesium	200 mg	200	225	250	300	350	375	375
Iron	7 mg	7	8	8	9	10	10	10
Zinc	7 mg	7	8	9	10	12	14	15
Chromium	35 mcg	35	37	40	43	45	50	50
Manganese	1.5 mg	2	2.5	3	3.5	4	4.5	5
Selenium	30 mcg	33	37	40	43	47	50	50

supplement (also containing magnesium) each day. These can be crushed and sprinkled on food or taken in a milky drink.

Are there any dangers with supplementing children?
Children tend to be more susceptible to vitamin toxicity than adults. As with all nutrients it is the dosage that counts. However, the doses listed on p.141 are well within any potentially toxic limits for even the most sensitive child and are, therefore, non-toxic. The fat soluble vitamins A, D and E store in the body and, therefore, can be more toxic if the intake is too high for many months. However, all of these are especially needed by children and are so often deficient. The vegetarian form of vitamin A, beta-carotene, is non-toxic and can, therefore, be taken in large amounts without any need for concern.

Special needs at adolescence
From the ages of ten to fifteen sexual development is in full swing. In both girls and boys this creates an extra demand for nutrients and the need for good nutrition. Especially important are vitamin B_6, zinc, vitamin A and essential fatty acids. Boys are more dependent on adequate zinc supply. Zinc is found in the highest concentration in the testes. It is thought that boys may stop growing as fast as girls in puberty precisely because of inadequate zinc intake, with what zinc is available being channelled towards sexual maturation rather than growth. So it is vital to ensure an ideal intake of these nutrients, as well as adequate protein.

NUTRIENTS AGAINST AGEING

Nutritional needs increase later in life as the ability to absorb declines. The loss of sense of taste (so often a result of zinc deficiency) can also lead to diets high in meat and dairy produce and other strong tasting foods, rather than fruit and vegetables. In women, calcium is most important since the decline in oestrogen levels, which bring on the menopause, also causes poor utilization of calcium. The result is osteoporosis, or porous bones, which is a major cause for backache and fractures in the elderly. 1,000 mg of calcium is needed daily to help keep the bones strong yet, according to one survey, 73 per cent of women don't even get half this amount!

The immune system also becomes less efficient later in life, making older people more prone to infections. Vitamins A, C, and E, as well as zinc, calcium and magnesium, are all important for boosting immune power. The mineral selenium has been shown in animals to substantially increase lifespan.

Premature loss of memory and mental function is one of the most serious problems among the elderly. No less than one in seven people over 65 are classified as senile. One of the causes for premature senility is aluminium poisoning. This is usually the result of aluminium pots and pans, or taking antacids frequently — obviously this is to be avoided. Another cause is a drop in acetylcholine levels, an important neurotransmitter involved in memory. Vitamins B, and choline help to make more acetylcholine and often help those with premature senility.

ALLERGY TESTING

In the last few years deserved attention has been focused on allergies. While there are many sceptics who feel that allergies are all in the mind, there are as many allergics who will literally pass out, puff up, get sleepy, or even become neurotic, when they eat the smallest amount of the allergen (substance to which they react) even if they don't know they've eaten it.

What is an allergy
An allergy can be thought of as an unusual reaction to any substance. However, a detrimental reaction is not always an allergy. For instance, excess alcohol will always cause a

reaction, but that doesn't indicate allergy. However, headaches after eating wheat products may indicate that wheat is an allergen for that particular person. Some allergies appear to exist from birth, while the majority arise as a result of the regular exposure to a particular substace. These are called 'masked allergies' and are like addictions when relating to foods, since the person usually craves the food despite its detrimental effect.

Finding the allergens

If you suspect that you may have allergies but do not know to what, the first thing to do is a simple elimination diet. This involves eliminating the top 10 allergic substances, while not taking vitamin or mineral supplements which can hide the allergies. Since we mainly develop allergies to commonly eaten foods, it is important to plan your dietary requirements carefully before starting in elimination diet.

Before beginning, keep a record of all symptoms for one week before starting the diet, prepare and purchase the foods that will be required, and follow the diet completely for 30 days. At the onset take a good dose of Epsom Salts in water and repeat in four hours if the result is not satisfactory (a good dose is 3–4 teaspoons).

Avoid the following:

1	Milk	7	All food colourings
2	Wheat	8	All additives
3	Eggs	9	Tobacco
4	Corn	10	All medication (discuss
5	Sugar		with doctor)
6	Citrus fruits	11	Supplements

Foods that may be eaten are meat, fish and chicken (except pork products), all vegetables (except corn), nuts (except peanuts), fruit (except citrus fruit), and a little maple syrup or honey can be used as a sweetener. It is best to drink only herb teas, spring water and fruit juice.

If this diet produces a significant improvement in health, by the end of the 30 days, it is most likely that you are allergic to some of these substances. You can then reintroduce each substance into your diet, one item per day, and make a note of any reaction. In this way it is often possible to find obvious allergies. However, if you do not have any clear results you may benefit from a cytotoxic or intradermal allergy test.

Intradermal allergy testing

As the name implies, intradermal allergy testing involves injecting tiny amounts of the suspected substance under your skin. This forms a small bubble, similar to having an inoculation. If you react to this substance the bubble increases in size within ten minutes. The advantage with this technique is that you can vary the concentration of the allergen, by diluting it further, and find what dilutions no longer induce an allergic reaction. This is useful for desensitizing the patient.

Cytotoxic allergy testing

The advantage of cytotoxic allergy testing is that you can test some 50 substances from one blood sample. The blood is introduced into an environment which contains the suspected food, and the way in which the cells in the blood react is carefully monitored using a powerful microscope. This technique depends largely on the skill of the technician who must carefully observe the behaviour of leucocytes in the blood, which are involved in allergic responses. Depending on the severity of the allergy, the leucocytes become less active, change shape and can even rupture.

Treating allergies

Having identified your allergens there are basically three methods of treatment. The first is avoidance and rotation. For instance, if you found that you reacted strongly to dairy products, causing extreme abdominal pain and lethargy, you avoid milk products entirely for a two month period. After two months you could rotate milk products by having them once every four days, for another two months. After that period you may be able to tolerate milk products every other day, or even every day provided your intake was not excessive. There are no hard and fast rules about how long each stage must be carried out, or how much of the substance you will eventually be able to tolerate. That varies so much from individual to individual.

Desensitization is another treatment which involves finding specific dilutions of the allergen, through intradermal injection, that no longer cause a reaction. In case you're thinking that the allergic reaction simply disappears because the dilution no longer contains enough of the allergen, it is quite common for no reaction to take place at a dilution of, for example, 1 part in 1000, and for a reaction to occur at a dilution of 1 part in 10,000. There seem to be particular levels which are desensitizing dosages. These are then given on a daily basis as drops under the tongue to desensitize the person against that particular food. Most allergy specialists recommend avoiding the substance during desensitization if the allergy is severe; however, minor allergens can be tolerated while taking the drops.

Vitamin and mineral supplementation is also highly effective for treating allergies especially since most chronic allergics have poor absorption and restrictive diets, and are therefore prone to deficiences. Some nutritionists believe that allergies are caused solely by vitamin and mineral deficiences, while on the other hand, some allergy specialists believe that supplementation merely hides the underlying allergy. I believe that we all have underlying intolerances to different substances; however, it is only when our health is less than perfect that these intolerances become a major problem. So often, improving someone's nutrition, helping them sort out their mental and emotional problems, and getting regular exercise, makes a considerable difference to the severity of allergic responses.

BUILDING YOUR VITAMIN PROGRAMME

On the basis of the questionnaire in previous sections you may already have some idea of the nutrients you could probably benefit from. By answering the Which Vitamins? questionnaire, make a list of the vitamins which you were most likely lacking. From the Which Minerals? chart or from a Hair Mineral Analysis, make a list of the nutritional minerals you suspect to be deficient.

Choosing the right supplements

Of course, buying each vitamin or mineral supplement separately always works out more expensive and awkward if it means taking a dozen vitamins a day. So it is usually best to find one or two supplement formulas which contain everything you need in the right doses. Here are some tips to help you find the right supplement for you.

The hidden ingredients

Contrary to many people's beliefs, a vast number of supplements contain the same additives, preservatives, colourings, and sugar that have helped our health to deteriorate in the first place. The best rule of thumb is to buy only those supplements which clearly declare all their ingredients, and use only natural excipients. (Excipients are the materials used to bind, coat, lubricate or fill the tablet.) The best excipients to use are calcium phosphate, magnesium stearate, yeast, kelp, and gum acacia. If any others are used make sure you know what they are.

B complex

If you show deficiency symptoms of any B vitamin it is wise to take a B complex tablet, as well as the individual B vitamin, which contains all the major B vitamins. It is also important to make sure that there is an effective quantity of each B vitamin. As a rule of thumb, a B complex should contain at least 25 mg of B_1, B_2, B_3, B_5, and B_6. A good B complex also contains 25 mg of choline, inositol, PABA, as well as 10 mcg of B_{12}, 50 mcg of folic acid, and biotin.

Multivitamins

There are a number of multivitamins on the market which contain insignificant quantities of vitamins and minerals, which could never produce any significant change in one's health. A multivitamin should contain at least 25 mg of the five major B vitamins, 5000 IUs of vitamin A, 400 IUs of vitamin D, 100 IUs of vitamin E, and 250 mg of vitamin C.

Multiminerals

Most minerals are not absorbable when supplied as a pure mineral. They must therefore be bound to another substance to make, for example, calcium carbonate, zinc sulphate, or potassium orotate. Depending on the mineral, different binding agents are used to maximize absorption. However, whatever the binding agent it is important to make sure you know the dosage of the mineral in question and not the dosage of the mineral plus binder. For example, a supplement advertized as zinc orotate 50 mg may only contain 5 mg of zinc. This can be very misleading, so most conscientious manufacturers also state the 'elemental value' or the actual amount of the nutritional mineral.

Unless you know, from a hair mineral analysis, that you are low in copper, it is best to avoid multiminerals which contain copper, since copper excess through copper water pipes is extremely common and supplementing this mineral could make the situation worse. Another point to watch out for is multiminerals containing selenium. Most forms of selenium are only usable when taken without food or other supplements. It is therefore best to supplement selenium separately. A good multimineral should contain at least 200mg of calcium, 150mg of magnesium, 10mg of potassium, 5mg of zinc, 5mg of manganese, 2mg of iron, and 20mcg of chromium.

Building your vitamin programme

The following programmes form safe and effective programmes suitable for everybody. Depending on your state of health and signs of deficiency you may wish to add individual nutrients to these programmes. For instance, if you live in a polluted area it would be wise to add the detoxifying nutrients outlined earlier, and if you have PMS, you may wish to double your dosage of B_6 and zinc. The next section, outlines possible programmes for common diseases. However, please note that everybody's needs are different, and no one programme can be right for everyone.

	COMPREHENSIVE PROGRAMME	SUPER PROGRAMME
	These programmes ensure against common nutritional deficiencies.	These programmes are designed for those under stress, with deficiency symptoms, or after extra energy and performance.
FOR MEN	1 × MULTIVITAMIN 1 × VITAMIN C 1000mg 1 × MULTIMINERAL	1 × MULTIVITAMIN 2 × VITAMIN C 1000mg 1 × MULTIMINERAL 1 × E 500 IU*
FOR WOMEN	1 × MULTIVITAMIN 1 × VITAMIN C 1000mg 1 × MULTIMINERAL	1 × MULTIVITAMIN 2 × VITAMIN C 1000mg 1 × MULTIMINERAL

* If you have high blood pressure or are a possible candidate for heart disease, it is wise to build up to this level of vitamin E, by taking up to 400 IU for one month, and then taking 600 IU for the next month. Provided vitamin E is increased in this way it is extremely beneficial up to 2000 IUs.

	COMPREHENSIVE PROGRAMME	SUPER PROGRAMME
		1 × B COMPLEX
		1 × B$_6$ 100mg + ZINC 10mg
FOR CHILDREN (Every other day for under 5s)	1/2 × MULTIVITAMIN	1 × MULTIVITAMIN
	1/2 × VITAMIN C 1000mg	1 × VITAMIN C 1000mg
	1/2 × MULTIMINERAL	1 × MULTIMINERAL

How to take supplements

Supplements are best taken with food as this helps their absorption. Some nutritionists feel that it is important to take vitamins C and B, two or three times a day, as excess is readily excreted. However, most of the time the body will take what it needs, and I therefore recommend taking all supplements with breakfast, unless you have difficulty digesting and absorbing nutrients. Vitamin E and iron compete for absorption, so if your ability to absorb is poor, take extra E and iron six hours apart from each other. Selenium supplements should also be taken separately from food or other supplements.

NUTRITION PROGRAMMES FOR COMMON DISEASES

Most of the conditions covered in this chapter are quite serious and if you suffer from these you may like to seek the advice of a local nutritionist. The Institute for Optimum Nutrition, 5 Jerdan Place, London SW6 1BE produce a list of nutrition consultants (£1). Wherever possible, I have stated the exact dosage of each nutrient. However, I refer to multivitamins, multiminerals and B complexes assuming those you select contain the levels of nutrients described in the last chapter.

Unless stated otherwise, the best diet to follow is based upon the recommendations throughout this book, with particular emphasis on special dietary recommendations.

Nutrition programme for hypoglycaemics and diabetics

Supplements   1 × Multivitamin
                   2 × Vitamin C 1000mg
                   3 × Multimineral giving at least 20mg zinc, 20mg manganese, 100mcg chromium

Diet   Avoid all sugar and refined grains. Eat high levels of protein and vegetables. Take regular exercise.

Nutrition programme for a healthy heart

Supplements   1 × Multivitamin
                   3 × Vitamin C 1000mg
                   1 × Vitamin E 500 IU (double after one month)
                   1 × Multimineral
                   1 × Selenium 50mcg
                   1 × B_6 100mg
                   2 × MaxEPA capsules (or 2 teaspoons of cod liver oil)

Diet   Avoid sugar, salt, excess fats, red meat, and smoking. Take regular exercise.

Nutrition programme for those with indigestion

Supplements   1 × Digestive Enzymes with Betaine Hydrochloride before each meal
                   1 × Vitamin C 1000mg
                   2 × Vitamin A 10,000 IU

       1 × Multivitamin
       2 × Multimineral giving at least 400mg
         calcium
       300mg magnesium
       1 × B complex

Diet   Eat plenty of alkaline forming foods, avoid citrus fruit, and watch food combinations.

Nutrition programme for chronic constipation

Supplements   3 × Vitamin C 1000mg
              1 × Multivitamin
              1 × Multimineral
              4 × Vitamin A 5000 IU and vitamin D
                 400 IU
              2 × Vitamin E 500 IU

Diet   Eat plenty of high fibre foods, avoid bread and red meat, and get regular exercise for the stomach muscles.

Nutrition programme for allergies

Supplements   2 × Multivitamins
              3 × Vitamin C 1000mg
              4 × Vitamin B_6 100mg + zinc 10mg
              1 × Manganese 50mg
              2 × B_3 100mg

Diet   Follow the elimination diet.

Nutrition programme for a healthy mind (high histamine type)

Supplements   2 × Vitamin C 1000mg
              2 × Multimineral
              3 × B_6 100mg + zinc 10mg
              1 × Manganese 50mg

Diet Avoid large quantities of greens and spinach, and keep protein intake low.

Nutrition programme for a healthy mind (low histamine type)

Supplements
$2 \times$ Multivitamin
$2 \times$ Vitamin C 1000mg
$5 \times$ B$_3$ 100mg
$1 \times$ Folic acid 1000mcg
$2 \times$ Multimineral
$1 \times$ B$_6$ 100mg + zinc 10mg
$2 \times$ Manganese 50mg

Diet Eat plenty of protein.

Nutrition programme for arthritis

Supplements
$2 \times$ Vitamin C 1000mg
$2 \times$ Multivitamin
$1 \times$ Multiminerals
$4 \times$ Detox formula
$1 \times$ B$_5$ 500mg

Diet Avoid wheat, sugar, salt, coffee, and stress. Check copper levels with hair mineral analysis. Get regular exercise.

Nutrition programme for premenstrual tension

Supplements
$2 \times$ Vitamin C 1000mg
$1 \times$ Multivitamin
$1 \times$ Multimineral
$3 \times$ B$_6$ 100mg + zinc 10mg
$1 \times$ B complex

Diet Avoid excess wheat, sugar, salt, coffee.

Nutrition programme for cancer

Supplements   10 × Vitamin C 1000mg
6 × Vitamin A 5000 IU
2 × Multivitamin
2 × Multimineral
1 × Selenium 50mcg
1 × Potassium 99mg

Diet   Avoid red meat and high protein diet. Eat plenty of fruit and vegetables, and drink plenty of water.

Nutrition programme for nerves and insomnia

Supplements   1 × Vitamin C 1000mg
1 × Multivitamin
1 × B complex
2 × B_6 100mg + zinc 10mg
2 × Multimineral (before bed)

Diet   Avoid all adrenal stimulants such as coffee, strong tea, salt, sugar, and cigarettes. Get regular exercise.

Nutrition programme for exhaustion

Supplements   2 × Vitamin C 1000mg
1 × Multivitamin
4 × B complex
2 × Vitamin E 500 IU
1 × Multimineral

Diet   Avoid all adrenal stressors, e.g. salt, sugar, coffee, strong tea, and refined grains. Eat plenty of salads.

Nutrition programme for multiple sclerosis

Supplements   1 × Vitamin C 1000mg
3 × B complex
1 × Multivitamin

2 × Evening primrose oil 500mg
2 × Vitamin E 500 IU
1 × Multimineral
1 × B_6 100mg + zinc 10mg

Diet   Avoid red meat and all gluten-containing grains.

Nutrition programme for acne and skin problems

Supplements   3 × Vitamin C 1000mg
3 × B_6 100mg + zinc 10mg
4 × Vitamin A 5000 IU
1 × Multivitamin
1 × Multimineral

Diet   Avoid acid diet, sugar, cigarettes, excess fats. Drink plenty of water and take regular exercise.

BIBLIOGRAPHY

Adams and Murray, *Minerals: Kill or Cure*, Larchmont Books, 1978.

Airola, *How to Get Well*, Health Plus, 1979.

Ballentine, *Diet and Nutrition*, Himalayan International Institute, 1978.

Brandt, *The Grape Cure*, Ehret Literature Publishing Company.

Buchinger, *About Fasting*, Thorsons Publishers, 1977.

Clinkard, *Eating for Health*, Whitcombe and Tombs, 1973.

Croft, *Relief from Arthritis*, Thorsons Publishers, 1979.

Davies, *Let's Eat Right to Keep Fit*, Unwin Paperbacks, 1979.

Fulder, *Ginseng*, Thorsons Publishers, 1976.

Kalita and Williams, *Physician's Handbook on Orthomolecular Medicine*, Keats Publishing Inc., 1977.

Newbold, *Meganutrients for Your Nerves*, Berkley Books, New York, 1978.

Nutrition Search Inc., *Nutrition Almanac*, McGraw Hill, 1975.

McNaught and Callander, *Illustrated Physiology*, Churchill Livingstone, 1963.

Moore and Lappe, *Diet for a Small Planet*, Ballantine Books, New York.

Pauling, *Vitamin C, Common Cold and Flu*, Berkley Books, New York, 1981.

Pfeiffer, *Mental and Elemental Nutrients*, Keats Publishing Inc., 1975.

Prevention Magazine, *Complete Book of Vitamins*, Rodale Press, 1977.

Sheldon, *Superior Nutrition*, Dr Sheldon's Health School, 1951–76.

Shears, *Nutritional Science and Health Education*, Downfield Press, 1976.

Shears, *Orthomolecular Nutrition*, Keats Publishing Inc., 1978.

Stone, *The Healing Factor*, Grosset and Dunlap, 1972.

Trum and Hunter, *Yogurt and Kefir*, Keats Publishing Inc., 1973.

Williams, *Biological Individuality*, John Wiley and Sons, Inc., 1956.
Wright, *The Nutrition Handbook*, Green Press.
Here's Health Magazine.

Many thanks to all these authors for their dedication to a healthier humanity.

USEFUL ADDRESSES

Association of Nutrition Consultants can refer you to a nutrition consultant in your area. They publish a directory of qualified nutrition consultants trained at the Institute for Optimum Nutrition. To receive the directory please send £1 to ANC, Maryland, Croft Road, Hastings, East Sussex.

Foresight provides information and personal advice on the importance of pre-conceptual care and nutrition. For more details send an SAE to Foresight, The Old Vicarage, Church Lane, Witley, Godalming, Surrey GU8 5PN.

Health+Plus vitamin company produce good quality vitamin supplements available by mail order. For more details ring or write to Health+Plus Ltd, Health+Plus House, Chinnor, Oxon OX9 4EZ (Tel: 0844 52098).

Hyperactive Children's Support Group offer help and advice for the families of hyperactive children. Please send an SAE to HACSG, 71 Whyke Lane, Chichester, West Sussex PO19 2LD.

Institute for Optimum Nutrition offers courses and personal consultations with trained nutritionists, including Patrick Holford. They also publish a quarterly magazine, *Optimum Nutrition*, available to ION members. For more details send an SAE to I.O.N., 5 Jerdan Place, London SW6 1BE (Tel: 071-381 5698).

INDEX

The Whole Health Manual

The drastic changes that have taken place in our lifestyle in the last fifty years have resulted in an alarming increase in the incidence of degenerative diseases such as arthritis, heart disease and cancer. The pace of life is very much quicker, the air we breathe is polluted and the food we eat has changed, but it is possible to combat these hazards and maintain good health.

The answers are in this comprehensive easy-to-read guide to nutrition.

Patrick Holford explains how our bodies work, and he shows how to balance your diet to suit your own individual needs. He also presents an easy-to-use and accurate system for calculating your personal vitamin programme.

Patrick Holford is an influential force in the world of nutritional therapy. He writes and lectures, and runs regular courses on nutrition.

HEALTH

UK £3.99
AUS $10.95 rrp
USA $6.95
CAN $7.95

ISBN 0-7225-1682-7

9 780722 516829